# Short Textbook of Prosthetics and Orthotics

# Short Textbook of Prosthetics and Orthotics


*Author*

**R Chinnathurai** MBBS, D Phys. Med.
Professor of Physical Medicine
Madras Medical College, Chennai, India
&
Head of the Institution
Govt. Institute of Rehabilitation Medicine
KK Nagar, Chennai

*Co-authors*

**P Sekar** MBBS, MD (Ped), DCH
Professor of Pediatrics
Institute of Child Health
Madras Medical College, Chennai

**M Ramaa Kumar** MS, FRCS
Consultant Surgeon
Mu. Va. Hospital, Chennai
Vadapalani Multispecialty Hospital, Chennai

**K Nithya Manoj** MBBS, D Phys. Med.
Civil Assitant Surgeon
Tutor in Physical Medicine
Govt. Institute of Rehabilitation Medicine
KK Nagar, Chennai

**C Senthil Kumar** B Tech, M Tech
Postgraduate Trainee
Uppsala University, Uppsala
Sweden


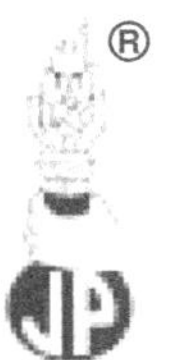


**JAYPEE BROTHERS MEDICAL PUBLISHERS (P) LTD**

Chennai • St Louis (USA) • Panama City (Panama) • New Delhi • Ahmedabad
Bengaluru • Hyderabad • Kochi • Kolkata • Lucknow • Mumbai • Nagpur

*Published by*

Jitendar P Vij

**Jaypee Brothers Medical Publishers (P) Ltd**

***Corporate Office***

4838/24 Ansari Road, Daryaganj, **New Delhi** - 110002, India, Phone: +91-11-43574357, Fax: +91-11-43574314

***Registered Office***

B-3 EMCA House, 23/23B Ansari Road, Daryaganj, **New Delhi** - 110 002, India
Phones: +91-11-23272143, +91-11-23272703, +91-11-23282021
+91-11-23245672, Rel: +91-11-32558559, Fax: +91-11-23276490, +91-11-23245683
e-mail: jaypee@jaypeebrothers.com, Website: www.jaypeebrothers.com

***Offices in India***

- **Ahmedabad**, Phone: Rel: +91-79-32988717, e-mail: ahmedabad@jaypeebrothers.com
- **Bengaluru**, Phone: Rel: +91-80-32714073, e-mail: bangalore@jaypeebrothers.com
- **Chennai**, Phone: Rel: +91-44-32972089, e-mail: chennai@jaypeebrothers.com
- **Hyderabad**, Phone: Rel:+91-40-32940929, e-mail: hyderabad@jaypeebrothers.com
- **Kochi**, Phone: +91-484-2395740, e-mail: kochi@jaypeebrothers.com
- **Kolkata**, Phone: +91-33-22276415, e-mail: kolkata@jaypeebrothers.com
- **Lucknow**, Phone: +91-522-3040554, e-mail: lucknow@jaypeebrothers.com
- **Mumbai**, Phone: Rel: +91-22-32926896, e-mail: mumbai@jaypeebrothers.com
- **Nagpur**, Phone: Rel: +91-712-3245220, e-mail: nagpur@jaypeebrothers.com

***Overseas Offices***

- **North America Office, USA,** Ph: 001-636-6279734
  e-mail: jaypee@jaypeebrothers.com, anjulav@jaypeebrothers.com
- **Central America Office, Panama City, Panama,** Ph: 001-507-317-0160
  e-mail: cservice@jphmedical.com
  Website: www.jphmedical.com

***Short Textbook of Prosthetics and Orthotics***



*First Edition:* **2010,** Reprint: 2026

ISBN 978-81-8448-819-7

*Typeset at* JPBMP typesetting unit

*Printed in India*

# Preface

Physical Medicine and Rehabilitation has always been a reign unexplored by most medical professionals and paramedical personnel. There is a lacunae in the realm of prescribing an appropriate and most useful prosthesis and orthosis to the needy disabled population.

This book *Short Textbook of Prosthetics and Orthotics* is meant to fill in the lacunae and provide sufficient information to medical professionals, prosthetic and orthotic technicians, physiotherapists, general practitioners, orthopedicians and sports physicians.

We have simplified the text with only brief technical details with specific emphasis laid on certain common disabling conditions.

The contents have been dealt with under the heads of medical diagnosis so as to ensure that the readers can refer to it as and when a patient approaches and a prescription is needed.

The pace of growth in the field of Prosthetics and Orthotics is very fast and hence is the variety of technology available for the patient.

We have laid emphasis on the technology that is widely available and used, and the global trends in the field have been dealt within appropriate Chapters.

We regard it as a reward if the book encourages further study of Orthotics and Prosthetics. We also welcome constructive criticism for improvement.

**R Chinnathurai**

# Acknowledgments

I express my deep sense of gratitude to my mentor Dr IS Shanmugam, Former Director, Govt. Institute of Rehabilitation Medicine for infusing interest in Physical Medicine and Rehabilitation during and after my student years with him.

I also thank my friends, colleagues and co-authors – Dr P Sekar and Dr M Ramaa Kumar for their beckoning inspiration and contribution in authoring this book. Their contribution on surgical aspects of amputee rehabilitation and comprehensive rehabilitation of pediatric population has enriched the scope of the title. Also I thank my student and co-author Dr K Nithya Manoj for her efforts to bring this work into its final shape of a book.

The technical aspects of prosthesis and latest developments in the field of biotechnology included in the book are a valuable contribution of the co-author, Mr C Senthil Kumar and I extend my thanks to him for his helping hand.

I deeply appreciate the work of Dr Selwyn J Kumar and Dr R Rajkumar for their active suggestions for improvement of the book.

I thank Mrs N Vijaya for the data entry work and my cousin Mr K Rajendran for scanning of pictures and illustrations for the book.

My endeavors would have been lost in the wood but for the continuous support and encouragement of the publishers M/s Jaypee Brothers Medical Publishers (P) Ltd and I pay my sincere thanks for their support.

Last but not the least, the book has seen the light of the day only with the affection and endurance of my wife, Mrs Malarkodi Chinnathurai.

# Contents

## SECTION I: PROSTHESIS



## SECTION II: ORTHOSIS

# Section I

# PROSTHESIS

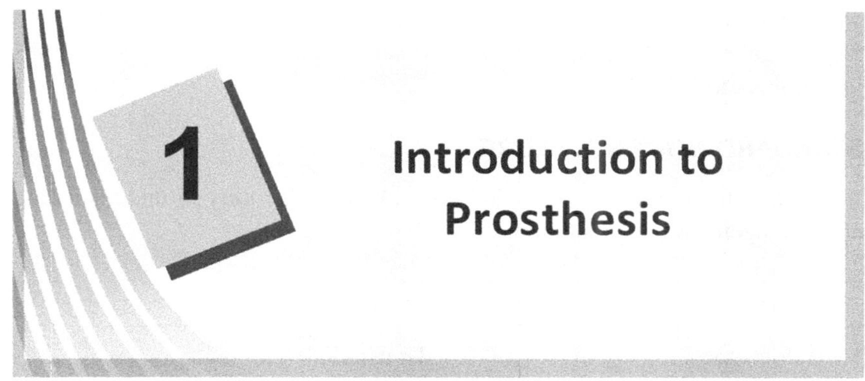

# 1 Introduction to Prosthesis

## A PROSTHESIS IS DEFINED AS ARTIFICIAL REPLACEMENT OF A PART OR WHOLE OF A LOST LIMB

Removal of a part or whole of a limb is called amputation. Amputations are done when all other modalities are explored, evaluated and rejected and removal of the limb is considered as the best solution for the patient.

A few milestones in the history of amputation surgery are as follows:

First prosthesis was given to Hegistratus in 484 BC who was imprisoned, chained at ankle and was awaiting death penalty. At his attempt to escape, he cut his foot and after wound healing he started using a wooden leg.

Hippocrates in fourth century BC reported about ligatures which was reintroduced by Ambrose Pare, a French military surgeon in 1529. Pare also introduced the Elbow disarticulation. He is called as the founder of *Modern*

### Principles of Amputation

First hip disarticulation was done by William Kerr of England in 1774.

Tarso metatarsal disarticulation was done by Lisfranc's, a French surgeon in 1815.

Disarticulation of ankle by James Symes in Edinburgh surgeon in 1843.

Antiseptic technique was introduced by Lord Lister in 1867.

Myoplasty was introduced by Burgess in 1956.

Immediate postoperative prosthesis was first fitted by Michael Berlemont in 1958.

Canadian hip disarticulation prosthesis was designed at Sunny Brook Hospital Toronto in 1954.

In 1955 Canadian Syme's prosthesis designed at the same hospital.

SACH foot was introduced by University of California in 1955.

In India first artificial limb center was started in Defense Medical College, Pune. Following that artificial limb center was started in Madras in the year 1965.

The field was extensively developed by Prof. M Natarajan, Prof. IS Shanmugam, Prof. K Janardhanam and others and achieved the present status in Tamil Nadu.

## STANDARD NOMENCLATURE

A standard nomenclature is needed for a global uniformity in understanding and management of amputations.

| | *Old terminology* | *Current terminology* |
|---|---|---|
| 1. | Below elbow | Transradial |
| 2. | Above elbow | Transhumeral |
| 3. | Below knee | Transtibial |
| 4. | Above knee | Transfemoral |
| 5. | Symes | Ankle disarticulation |
| 6. | Hemi pelvectomy | Transpelvic |

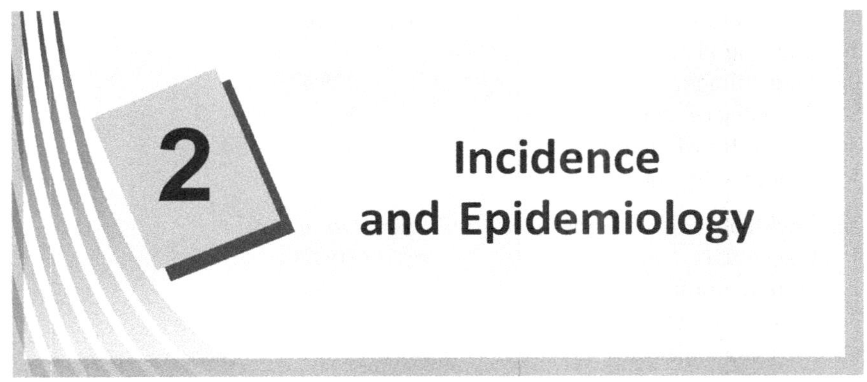

# 2 Incidence and Epidemiology

## CAUSES OF AMPUTATION

- **Trauma**
  a. Road traffic accident (RTA)/Train accidents
  b. Industrial accidents
  c. Fracture complications
  d. Burns–Thermal, electrical and chemical.
- **Vascular**
  a. Thromboangiitis obliterans
  b. Arteriosclerosis-Senile and diabetic
  c. Frost bite.
- **Infections**
  a. Leprosy
  b. Actinomycosis
  c. Filariasis
  d. Gas gangrene.
- **Tumors–Malignant**
  a. Bone—Osteosarcoma
  b. Soft tissue—Fibrosarcoma
- **Congenital Limb Deficiency**

## INCIDENCE

Most of the amputations are done in lower limb. Ratio of upper and lower limb amputation is 1: 4.9.

The incidences of common *upper limb amputations* are:

| | |
|---|---|
| 1. Transradial | 57% |
| 2. Transhumeral | 23% |
| 3. Wrist disarticulation | 7% |
| 4. Elbow disarticulation | 5% |
| 5. Shoulder disarticulation | 8% |

The incidences of common *lower limb amputations* are:

| | |
|---|---|
| 1. Transtibial | 59% |
| 2. Transfemoral | 35% |
| 3. Syme's amputation | 4% |
| 4. Hip disarticulation | 2% |
| 5. Knee disarticulation | 1% |

Study of cases reported for prosthesis fitting for 3 years (2003-06) at Government Institute of Rehabilitation Medicine KK Nagar, Chennai was undertaken to study the etiology of amputations in Indian scenario which showed that 67.8% of cases are traumatic, 12.4% are diabetic, 6.7% due to malignancy and 5% TAO. The etiology is further classified as follows (Fig. 2.1):

| *S.No.* | *Causes* | *Percentage %* |
|---|---|---|
| 1. | Congenital | 1.2 |
| 2. | Traumatic | |
| | a. Machinery accidents | |
| | – Road traffic accidents | 36.6 |
| | – Train traffic accidents | 9.5 |
| | – Industrial machinery | 6.7 |
| | – Agricultural machinery | 4.0 |
| | b. Other traumatic accidents | |
| | – Falls from height | 3.8 |
| | – Wall collapse | 1.9 |
| | – Assault | 0.5 |
| | – Blast | 0.2 |
| | – Electrocution | 3.6 |
| | – Fire cracker accidents | 1.0 |
| 3. | Systemic disease | |
| | – Diabetes mellitus | 12.4 |
| | – TAO | 5.0 |
| | – Malignancy | 6.7 |
| | – Leprosy | 1.9 |
| | – Infection and sepsis | 0.5 |

## CONCLUSION

- This study reveals that road traffic accident forms the major cause of amputation, in 36.6% in contrast to west where vascular problem is the main cause.

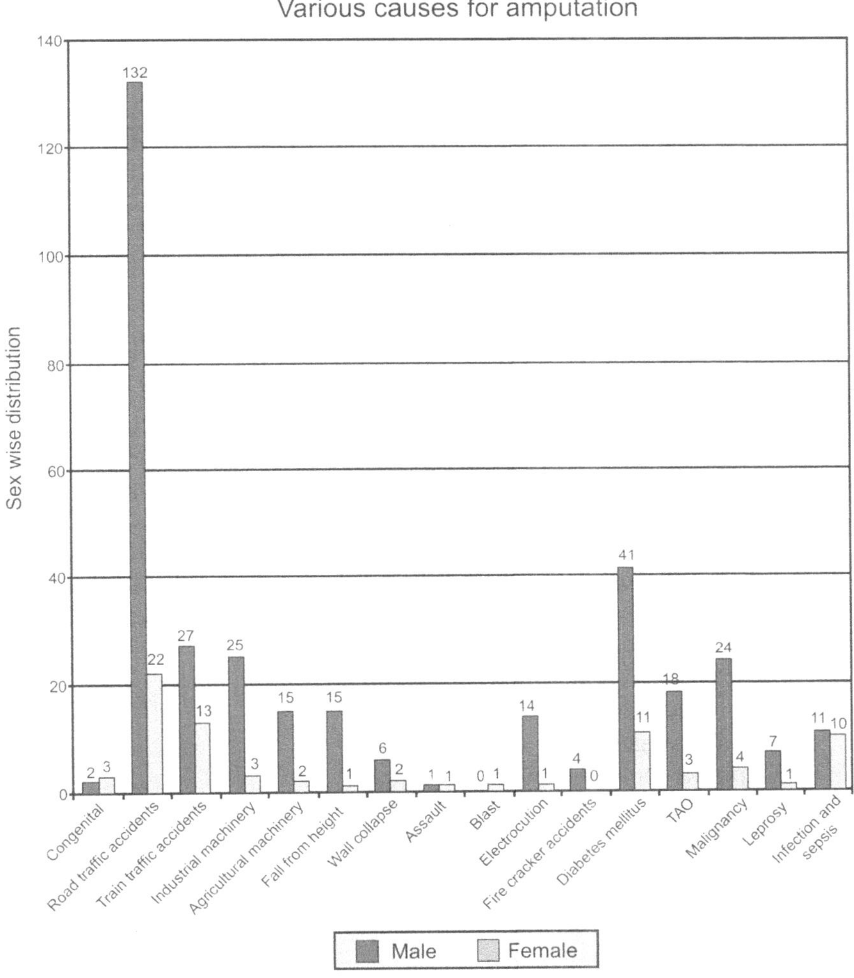


**Fig. 2.1:** Various causes for amputation

- The males in the age group of 20-40 are affected in large numbers. The average age of Indian amputees is lower than western amputees
- The proportion of injury of the upper limb to the lower limb is in the ratio of 1:5.
- The preventive measures to avoid the major cause, RTA have already been implemented by legislation and awareness campaigns. Special efforts may be taken to strengthen the implementation of the preventive measures.

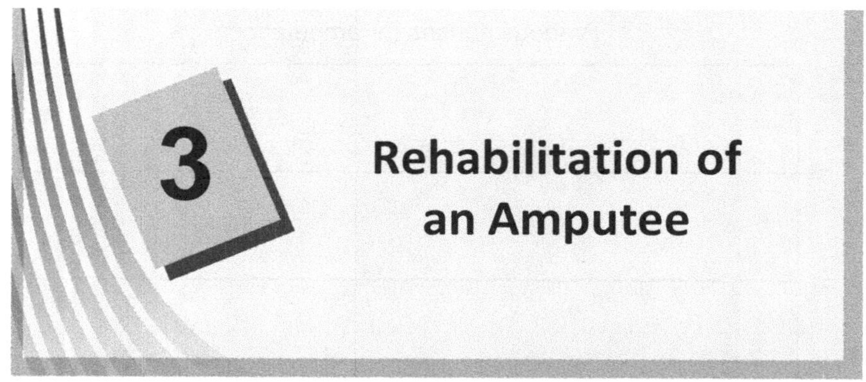


# 3 Rehabilitation of an Amputee

## INTRODUCTION

Rehabilitation is a process by which the patient's abilities are utilized to make him independent physically, mentally, socially and vocationally to make him lead a near normal life.

This is implemented by the rehabilitation team which is lead by the Physiatrist. The team is comprising of surgeon, related specialists, clinical psychologist, therapist and prosthetist.

The rehabilitation is done in the following stages:

1. Pre-amputation counseling
2. Amputation surgery
3. Acute post-amputation care
4. Preprosthetic training
5. Prosthetic fitting and training
6. Reintegration into community
7. Long-term follow-up.

## PRE-AMPUTATION COUNSELING

To prepare the patient physically and mentally for amputation and post-amputation period.

a. Communication involving patient, family to explain about need for surgery and outcome.
b. Communication between Surgeon, Physiatrist, prosthetist to discuss about level of amputation and prosthetic fitting.
c. Introductory session with patient regarding:
    1. Phantom limb sensation
    2. Prosthetic fittings
    3. Mode of fitting and training
    4. Time taken
    5. Cost expenditure

d. Demonstration by a trained volunteer and discussion between patient and volunteer.
e. Pre-rehabilitation exercise program involving:
   1. Other limbs
   2. Trunk muscles.

## AMPUTATION SURGERY

"AMBI" means around.
"PUTATIO" means trimming.
Separation by cutting of a terminal part of the body.

Amputation is done when all other modalities are explored, evaluated and rejected and the evidence suggests that the amputation is the best solution to the patient's plight.

**Amputation is to achieve:**
a. Most distal level with clinical condition
b. Well healed stump
c. Less functional loss
d. Less energy for ambulation with prosthesis.

**Amputation surgery includes:**
a. Removal of a part or whole limb to exclude pathology
b. Reconstruction to create a best possible stump.

### Types of Amputation

#### *Guillotine Amputation*

Emergency amputation is done as a life saving measure. It is the one done in case where primary healing unlikely to occur and amputation is done as low as possible to allow room for re-amputation. The bone, muscles and skin are cut at same level.

#### *Definite (Classical) Amputation*

One for which no further operative procedure is expected and prosthesis can be fitted to the patient.

#### *Revision Amputation*

Done in already amputated persons, e.g. guillotine amputation, childhood amputation etc to get good stump.

### Technique of Amputation

All elective amputation patient should be prepared properly and undergo local preparation of the part of surgery.

### Anesthesia

Local, regional, spinal and general anesthesia can be given. The choice of anesthesia depends on the general condition of the patient, expertise of anesthetist and patients choice.

### Tourniquet

No tourniquet is applied in patients with peripheral vascular disease. In all other cases wherever possible, pneumatic tourniquet can be used.

### Stump Flaps

Stump flaps should be mapped out prior to surgery. It is always better to have long flaps to start with and excess can be trimmed later if necessary. In vascular diseases, a long posterior flap is preferred to promote better healing of the wound.

### Bone

Bone level is marked prior to surgery. In transtibial amputation, the fibula is cut 1-3 cm above tibia. The tibia is beveled at 45 to 60 degrees. All the cut edges are filled and sculptured to get a round non-pointing end.

### Muscles

Muscles carry blood supply from deep to the fascia, skin, etc. So it should not be dissected from deep fascia or skin. Muscles can provide:

1. Padding at lower end
2. Provides stump control when fixed
3. Give proprioceptive feedback.

To achieve this the following surgical techniques are used.

a. *Myoplasty:* Attachment of opposite compartment muscles to each other and to the periosteum at the cut end of bone is called myoplasty.
b. *Myodesis:* The muscles and fascia are sutured directly to the bone through drill holes.

### Nerves

Proper care in handling of peripheral nerves is important to prevent future complication like stump neuroma.

a. Nerves are gently pulled and cut as high as possible and allowed to retract and bury in deeper tissues.
b. Nerve end can also be injected with neurolytic agents like phenol.
c. Nerve end can be buried in bone.
d. Nerve end can be enclosed by material like silicone.

### *Blood Vessels*

Blood vessels are isolated, ligated and cut to achieve hemostasis and a drain is put. Vacuum suction is preferred.

### *Wound Closure*

Wound is closed in layers with physiological tension neither too tight nor too loose.

### *Skin Closure*

Skin is closed by interrupted sutures rather than continuous suture.

### *Stump*

The residual part of limb left after amputation is called as Stump. The word ideal stump is not used nowadays as prosthesis can be given to any length of stump. In addition the length may be ideal for one prosthesis and not for other. Example in below elbow prosthesis the length of 8 inches is ideal for using body powered mechanical hand and long for electronically powered myoelectric hands. Hence the word good stump is better used.

**Good stump** is described as the one with the following features:

1. Proper length (size)
2. Proper shape (shape)
3. Skin is free (skin)
4. Scar is healthy and free (scar)
5. Muscles have good power (strength)
6. Joint should have full range of movement (no deformity)
7. No neuroma
8. No phantom sensation or pain.

### *Levels of Amputation*

Selection of surgical level for amputation is an important decision to be made for an amputee . Most of the time the pathology dictates the level of amputation. In malignancy, when local resection and chemotherapy is not advisable, amputation above proximal joint is advised. Viability of tissues determines the level in other cases. The level of amputation in vascular cases are mostly determined at operating rooms based on skin bleeding.

Lower limb amputations—named by the bones involved (transfemoral/ transtibial) and according to the length of the residual stump (very short, short, medium and long)—lower limb joint disarticulations (hip, knee, Syme's ankle disarticulations). Foot amputations are dealt within following Chapters (Fig. 3.1).

Upper limb amputations—includes different levels of amputation in arm (transhumeral) and forearm (transradial) and disarticulation of shoulder, elbow and wrist. Hand amputations can also be either transmetacarpal or transphalangeal (Fig. 3.2).

- *Transtibial Amputation*

Ideal length—Five inches from tibial tubercle
Minimum length—Two inches from tibial tubercle

a. Long transtibial—Junction of lower and middle 1/3 of tibia.
b. Standard transtibial—Junction of upper and middle 1/3 of tibia.
c. Short transtibial—In upper 1/3 of tibia
d. Ultrashort transtibial—Just below tibial tubercle

Healing rate improves inversely with stump length.

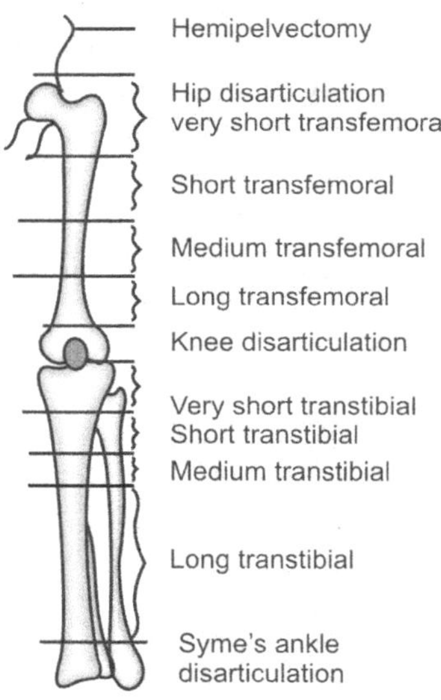


**Fig. 3.1:** Levels of amputation - lower limb

- *Transfemoral Amputation*

Ideal length—Ten inches from greater trochanter
Minimum length—Five inches from greater trochanter
Maximum length—Four inches from knee joint.

a. *Long above knee:* 55 to 75% of normal femur
b. *Medium above knee:* 35 to 55% of normal femur
c. *Short above knee:* Groin to 35% of normal femur
d. *Functional hip disarticulation:* Proximal to groin.

- *Knee Disarticulation*

Better than transfemoral amputation as prosthesis can be made with full distal weight bearing (end bearing).

- *Below Elbow Amputation*

Ideal length—Eight inches
Minimum length—Two inches
Maximum length—Three inches from wrist joint.

a. *Very short transradial:* 0 to 35% from medial epicondyle
b. *Short below elbow:* 35 to 55% from medial epicondyle
c. *Long below elbow:* 55 to 90% from medial epicondyle

- *Wrist disarticulation:* 90 to 100% from medial epicondyle

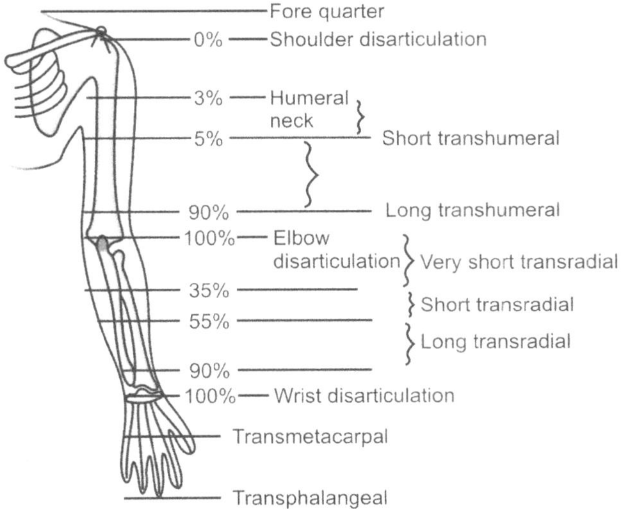


**Fig. 3.2:** Levels of amputation – Upper limb

- *Above Elbow Amputation*

Ideal length—Eight inches from acromion
Minimum length—Three inches from acromion

## POSTOPERATIVE CARE

The stump is maintained postoperatively by:

1. Soft dressing
2. Rigid dressing

3. Crepe bandaging
4. Controlled environment method
5. Immediate postoperative prosthetic fitting.

### Soft Dressing

*Advantages:*

1. Allows inspection of wound
2. Allows near normal Range of Movement.

*Disadvantages:*

1. Does not prevent contractures
2. Does not prevent trauma.

### Rigid Dressing

Postoperative rigid dressing in the form of plaster cast. It is called as Immediate Postoperative Rigid Dressing (IPORD).

*Advantages:*

1. Pain is decreased
2. Wound heals quickly
3. Edema is prevented
4. Prevent contractures
5. Protects from trauma.

*Disadvantages:*

1. Requires careful application
2. Wound inspection cannot be done.

### Crepe Bandaging

Bandaging is done like 'figure of 8'. It needs frequent rewrapping. This gives pressure from distal to proximal thus reducing hematoma and edema.

### Controlled Environment Method

It uses a machine that supplies bacteria free environment to the wound a with controlled humidity and temperature. This provides the perfect environment for primary healing.

### IPOPF

Immediate postoperative prosthetic fitting (IPOPF) can be done especially in children and clean traumatic ablations.

The main aims of postoperative care are:

1. Control of pain
2. Prevention of edema

3. Prevention of infection
4. Prevention of deformity/stiffness
5. Prevention of deep vein thrombosis
6. Improving muscle power.

*Control of pain:*

a. Narcotics /analgesics every 3 to 6 hours at least for 48 hours to a maximum of 5 days.
b. Switch on to a less potent narcotic or oral analgesics.
c. Local infiltration by a silastic catheter within or along nerves with local anesthetic 0.25 to 0.5%. Bupivacaine is administered by infusion pump at a rate of 2-3 ml/ hour for 72 hours can also be done.

*Prevention of edema:*

a. Passive ROM exercises.
b. Active exercise with muscle contraction helps in venous return and reduces edema.
c. *Creppe bandaging:* Like figure of 8 bandaging from distal to proximal. Frequent reapplication helps prevention of edema.
d. *Shrinkers:* Number of shrinkers are available.
   1. Provides good skin tolerance
   2. Provides pressure gradient from distal to proximal
   3. The elastic nature gives more comfort to patient by yielding to different sizes.

*Prevention of infection:* Proper wound care and with good antibiotic cover can prevent infections.

*Prevention of stiffness:*

a. Passive ROM exercise
b. Active mobilization exercise
c. Proper positioning
d. Early fitting of prosthesis.

*Prevention of deep vein thrombosis:*

a. Active and passive exercises
b. Elastic stockings
c. Elasto crepe bandages.

*Improving muscle power:*

a. Chest physiotherapy
b. Exercises to other limb
c. Exercises to upper limbs with intention to use for crutch walking and wheel chair mobility
d. Exercises to prevent general deconditioning.

*Postoperative Program in Amputee Training*

- **First day**
  1. Breathing exercise
  2. Proper positioning of limb and stump.
- **Second day**
  1. Sit up in bed
  2. Breathing exercise.
- **Third day**
  1. Drain removal
  2. Stump exercise
- **Fourth day**
  1. Standing with support/without support
  2. Crutch walking
- **Fifth to Seventh day**
  1. Suture removal
  2. Stump bandaging

## PREPROSTHETIC TRAINING

The preprosthetic training phase plays a main role in the successful outcome of prosthetic fitting and usage. This phase includes training in the following patterns:

1. Active ROM exercise
2. Proper positioning of stump
3. Muscle strengthening
4. Skin care
5. Crutch training
6. Wheel chair mobility
7. Self care
8. Patient and family education.

The final outcome on prosthetic usage depends on clinical condition, age and motivation during preprosthetic training.

## PROSTHETIC TRAINING

Person who receives new prosthesis or new model of prosthesis should undergo regular training program with a coordinated effort among physiotherapist, occupational therapist and prosthetist as per physiatrist advice.

The steps in prosthetic training includes:

1. *Prosthetic fitting:* Includes alignment check, pressure point relief, color matching, etc.

2. *Donning and doffing training:* For independence in self care activities
3. *Skin care training:* To avoid pressure ulcers, skin infections
4. *Gait training:* Includes weight bearing, weight transfers, stepping training, walking with or without assistive aids, stair climbing, etc.
5. *Maintenance of prosthesis:* Cleaning, maintaining and replacement of prosthesis.

## REINTEGRATION INTO COMMUNITY

- It has to be done gradually for weeks or months.
- Organized trips for shopping, recreation or a part time job should be done.
- *Day hospital rehabilitation program:* Patient participate in rehabilitation in hospital 6 hours per day 5 days a week and return home every evening and weekend. It is then followed by modified and restricted work and then made to return to normal work.

### Long-term Follow-up

During first year follow up is advised every three months and thereafter as and whenever required.

# 4 Problems in Stump

## ACUTE COMPLICATIONS

1. Hemorrhage/Hematoma
2. Stump edema
3. Wound gaping
4. Infections
5. Delayed wound healing
6. Deep vein thrombosis.

## DELAYED COMPLICATIONS

1. Skin complications:
   a. Increased sweating
   b. Skin ulceration
   c. Skin infections
   d. Adherent scar
   e. Dog ear
2. Bony complications:
   a. Osteoporosis
   b. Fracture of stump
   c. Stump osteophytes
   d. Osteomyelitis
   e. Overgrowth (in pediatric amputees).
3. Neuroma
4. Contracture
5. Muscle wasting
6. Phantom sensation
7. Phantom pain
8. Psychological problems.

## Skin Complications

### *Increased Sweating*

Increase in sweating is attributed to the following causes:

a. Toes and fingers takes active part in normal sweating. When they are lost it has to be compensated by remaining part of the limb and so more sweating is noted in stump.
b. Increase in energy requirement for ambulation results in increased metabolism and sweating.
c. Prosthesis prevents aeration of the limb.

### *Skin Ulceration*

Skin ulceration is the commonest problem in amputation stump. It may be due to:

a. *Anesthetic stump:* Unnoticed minor injuries with continued trauma in conditions like spina bifida, leprosy and diabetes leads to ulceration.
b. *Vascular diseases:* Deficient arterial perfusion augmented by pressure and infection leads to ulceration.
c. *Infection:* May be a primary infection of the stump or secondary to trauma or ischemia.
d. *Prosthetic causes:*
    i. Point of excess pressure leads to discomfort and ulceration
    ii. Not wearing socks
    iii. Faulty weight load or pressure at a particular point on stump
    iv. Stump volume reduced and descent into socket
    v. Pressure at lower end
    vi. Pressure over grafted skin.

### *Skin Infection*

Fungal infection secondary to perspiration is quite common. Infected hair follicles are treated by plucking of the infected hair and with antibiotics.

### *Adherent Scar*

Adherence of scar to underlying bone leads to concentration of stress during ambulation and may lead to ulceration.

### *Dog Ear*

Excess skin flap leads to formation dog ear. It can be avoided by proper mapping of flap before surgery and adequate trimming at the time of surgery.

## Bony Complications

1. *Osteoporosis:* Occurs commonly in case of ischial weight bearing prosthesis in transfemoral amputees and proximal weight bearing in Syme's amputation. The distal limb is not used for weight bearing and so results in osteoporosis.
2. *Fracture stump:* Can result due to trauma or may be a pathological fracture.
3. *Bone spurs:* Bone spurs is due to remaining periosteum left in the stump during surgery.
4. *Bony overgrowth:* In children amputation through long bone before bone maturity leads to increase in bone length later. It is due to endosteal and periosteal growth but skin does not grow much. So the bone end becomes pointed and pushes through skin.

   This complication is more common with below knee and above elbow amputations.

### *Bony Overgrowth*

This can be treated by:

a. Revision amputation
b. Angulation osteotomy in humerus
c. Capping of the stump with osteocartilagenous graft or plastic or silicone caps.

## Neuroma

Bulbous swelling at the cut end of the nerve is called a neuroma. The peripheral nerves, when transected, will attempt to regenerate by the growth of neurofibrills. In the absence of distal segment the neurofibrills at the stump grows into a disorganized mass and is known as neuroma.

Neuroma may be:

a. At major anatomical nerves
b. Cutaneous nerves in the scar tissue of stump at the lower end.

### *Prevention of Neuroma*

1. During surgery, the nerve is divided with sharp blade after gentle traction and allowed to retract proximally into soft tissues.
2. Crushing of the nerve end and cauterization to prevent regeneration.
3. Neurolytic agents like phenol or absolute alcohol into nerve end.
4. The severed nerve end is burried within bone.
5. Nerve end is enclosed in silicone cups.

### *Management of Neuroma*

Neuroma are painful only when subjected to pressure or shear. It can be managed by:

1. Pressure relief in prosthesis at the site of neuroma

2. Ultrasound/TENS (Transcutaneous Electrical Nerve Stimulation) over painful area
3. Injection of a local anesthetic with or without steroids.
4. Desensitization by tapping and kneading massage from early postoperative period
5. Surgical excision of neuroma.

## Phantom Sensation

The sensation of presence of the amputated part is called phantom sensation. First sensation to appear is:

a. To scratch the chin with the absent hand
b. To walk on missing leg.

Phantom sensation is absent in:

1. Congenital limb deficiencies
2. Amputation before 4 years
3. Patients with brain damage
4. Amputation of anesthetic limbs.

The reason for phantom sensation is explained by various theories of neuro-projection, like unablation of the cortical representation. The perceptions remembered by the cortex is said to produce phantom sensation. This also explains the reason why the deformity and problems before amputation continues as phantom sensation.

The sensation tends to disappear in duration of time. The last sensation to disappear is sensation from missing thumb or great toe.

## Phantom Pain

Painful, disagreeable sensation with strong paresthesia in absent limb is called as phantom pain. Phantom pain may be constant or intermittent. Phantom pain can be precipitated by:

a. Contact with painful stump
b. Trigger area anywhere in body
c. Urination/intercourse/angina
d. Emotional.

### *Theories of Pain*

*Central theory:*

a. The reticular activating system which has inhibitory control on pain gets initiated by sensory input from the limb. When large proportion of sensory fibers are destroyed by amputation it results in decreased inhibitory control by reticular activating system. The somatosensory projection areas develop a self sustaining neural activity thus causing pain.
b. Other theories involving thalamic, subthalamic and cortical involvement.

*Peripheral theory:* Spontaneous activity and painful sensory input is received by brain from the severed nerve site. Misinterpretation by the brain on the origin of the input of pain sensation.

*Psychological theory:* Emotional disturbance especially immediately after amputation, difficulty in using prosthesis or refusal to use prosthesis results in establishment of phantom pain.

### Types of Pain

1. Cramping pain like muscle spasm
2. Electric shock like pain that lasts for few seconds and it is lancinating and episodic
3. Burning pain felt throughout the stump and phantom limb
4. Squeezing pain.

*Ten-point program in treatment of phantom pain:*

1. Preoperative preparation of patient about phantom sensation that it is normal and is not harmful.
2. Postoperative examination of stump daily and advise to use the residual limb or stump.
3. Normal healing of stump is essential as infection and complications more likely to cause phantom sensation.
4. Massaging the stump and then toughening the skin by gentle pounding without damaging the skin.
5. Exercise the stump muscles with imaginary movement, e.g. pedaling an imaginary bicycle.
6. Provide prosthesis as soon as possible.
7. Local blocking agents like ethyl chloride spray; local procaine injection.
8. Physical therapy
9. Drugs:
   - Beta blockers
   - Anticonvulsants
   - Carbamazepine (most useful)
   - Phenytoin
   - Chlorpromazine
   - Antidepressants
   - Amitriptyline
   - Imipramine.
10. Surgical modalities:
    - Anterolateral cordotomy
    - Thalamic tracotomy
    - Subcortical neurectomy ablation of somatosensory cortex
    - Electrical stimulation of dorsal column of spinal cord.

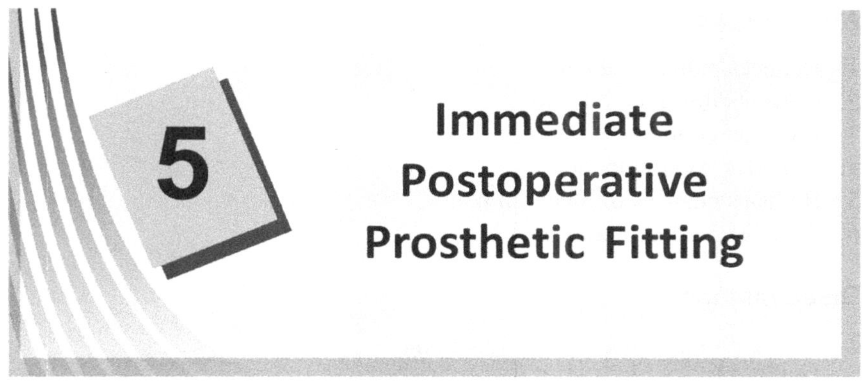

# 5 Immediate Postoperative Prosthetic Fitting

## IPOPF OR IPOP (IMMEDIATE POSTOPERATIVE PROSTHESIS)

Immediate postoperative fitting (IPOPF) was described by Berlemont in 1961 but Weiss popularized this technique in 1966.

A temporary prosthesis was applied in operating room at the conclusion of amputation. The most commonly used IPOP consists of a rigid plaster cast carefully molded to a patellar tendon bearing configuration to which pylon and foot is attached (Fig. 5.1).

Patient starts touch down weight bearing within 24-48 hours after surgery. Gradually weight bearing is increased with training in parallel bar and then with crutch and walkers.

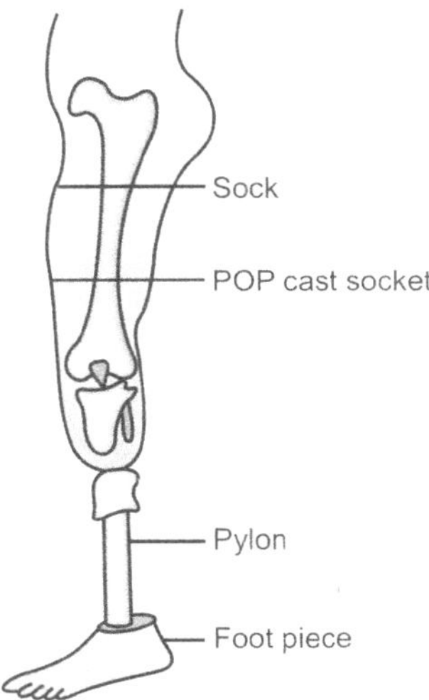


**Fig. 5.1:** Immediate Postoperative prosthetic fitting

## Advantages

1. Reduces pain and edema
2. Prevents muscular atrophy
3. Prevents contracture
4. Provides good motivation
5. Reduces chances of phantom pain
6. Speeds up rehabilitation.

## Disadvantages

1. Increased incidence of wound gaping
2. Delayed wound healing
3. Infection of wound.

## IMMEDIATE PROSTHESIS AFTER WOUND HEALING

- This is done after suture removal and wound healing.
- Immediate prosthesis after wound healing is safe.
- Because of problems with IPOP most surgeon advice temporary prosthesis after the wound is safe for touch down weight bearing.
  a. Harris (1977) advised prosthetic fitting after 7 to 10 days of amputation.
  b. Eraklis and Wheeler (1963) advised prosthetic fitting after 2-3 weeks.

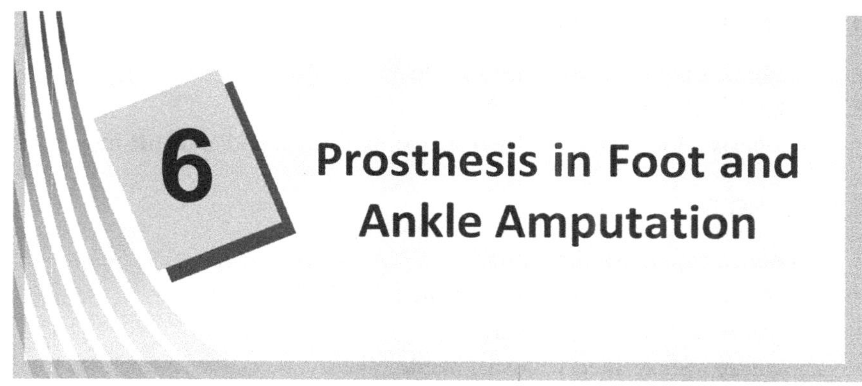

# 6 Prosthesis in Foot and Ankle Amputation

Foot amputation is done in various levels—from Syme's ankle disarticulation, calcaneo-tibial fusion (Boyd's and Pirogoffs), midtarsal amputation (Chopart's), tarsometatarsal disarticulation (Lisfranc's), transmetatarsal amputation to toe disarticulation (Fig. 6.1).

## LEVELS OF AMPUTATION IN FOOT AND ANKLE

1. Toe disarticulation
2. Transmetatarsal amputation
3. Tarsometatarsal disarticulation–Lisfranc
4. Midtarsal amputation–Chopart's
5. Calcaneotibial fusion–Boyd's, Pirogoff
6. Syme's amputation

## TOE DISARTICULATION

- No obvious functional loss.
- *Big toe:* Some difficulty in push off.
- *Prosthesis:* Toe filling of rubber, foam, wool as spacer and to prevent hyperextension of boot at toe-break.

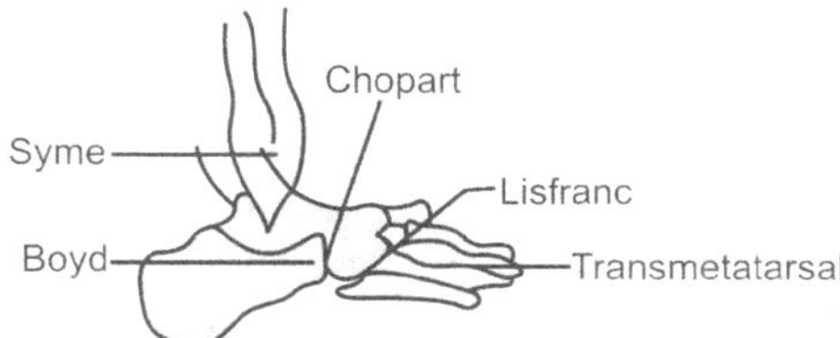


**Fig. 6.1:** Foot amputation

## TRANSMETATARSAL AMPUTATION

- Weight bearing metatarsal head are lost
- Push off difficult, foot flat difficult
- *Prosthesis:* Boot with long steel shank, metatarsal pad and stiff insole

## LISFRANC'S

- Tarsometatarsal disarticulation.
- Metatarsals and toes are removed and all tarsal retained.
- *Problems:* Equinus contracture.
- *Prosthesis:* Shoe filled with stiff insole.

## CHOPART'S AMPUTATION

- Calcaneum and talus retained.
- Remaining tarsals with metatarsal and toes removed.
- Equinus contracture is the complication
- Prosthesis:
  a. High collar shoe with toe filler
  b. Syme's model prosthesis.

**SYME'S AMPUTATION:** Syme's amputation is done in following ways (Fig. 6.2):

a. Original Syme's amputation
b. Two-stage Syme's amputation
c. Modified Syme's amputation

### Original Syme's Amputation

A thin layer of tibia with both malleoli are removed. The saw cuts in horizontal plane and parallel to ground. Heel pad is fixed by either of the following techniques:

a. External fixation with elastic straps
b. Internal fixation with K wire or thin Steinman pin.

### Two-stage Syme's Amputation

- Done in case of infective wound
- *1st stage:* Foot is removed and heel pad brought under tibia and sutured.
- *2nd stage:* After several weeks when infection is controlled both malleoli and front surface are removed. Heel pad fixed in lower end.

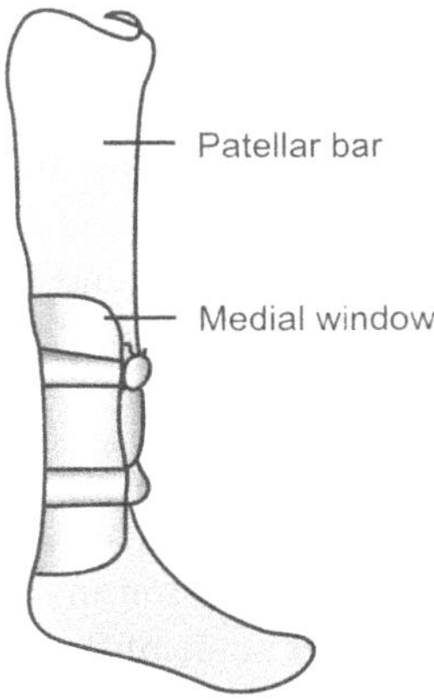


**Fig. 6.2:** Syme's prosthesis with medial opening

## Modified Syme's Amputation

The original technique was modified to get a less bulbous and more cosmetic stump.

a. Metaphyseal flare of tibia is removed.
b. Distal end of fibula is beveled and size of stump is reduced.

## Problems in Syme's Amputation

1. Misplaced heel pad
2. Sloping cut surface of tibia
3. Too small cross-section area of end bearing stump
4. Wobbly heel pad
5. Marginal gangrene of heel pad
6. Tender heel pad.

## Syme's Prosthesis

Syme's prosthesis should have end bearing pad for shock absorption.
Syme's prosthesis can be fabricated with the following types of weight bearing:

a. Full end bearing
b. More distal end bearing and less proximal PTB weight bearing
c. More proximal patellar tendon weight bearing and less end bearing.

Three types of Syme's prosthesis are described hereunder.

### *1. Conventional*

Conventional prosthesis is made of leather socket and wooden foot piece. Whole weight is end bearing. Most patients are unable to bear long time standing and distance walking.

### *2. Canadian Syme's Prosthesis*

This prosthesis consists of:

a. End bearing pad made of shock absorbing material
b. Patellar tendon bar partly bears weight
c. Medial window is given to pull bulbous end to the socket. It also provides suspension over malleoli.

### *3. Closed Expandable Syme's Prosthesis*

This is prescribed in cases with modified Syme's amputation, where the lower end is less bulbous and there is no need for any window.

The prosthesis has an inner layer made of flexible plastic or elastic attached to the inside of socket. It extends from distal end of socket proximally to a point where the diameter of proximal leg is equal with bulbous lower end. The inner layer stretches as the end of the stump inserted within the socket.

The advantages are better cosmesis and better suspension.

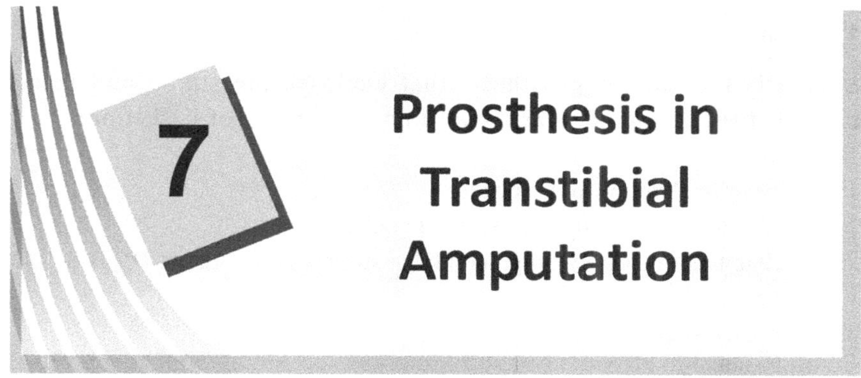

# 7 Prosthesis in Transtibial Amputation

Trans-tibial amputation accounts for 59% of lower limb amputation.
Ideal length of stump is 15 cm from tibial tubercle.
Minimum length is just below tibial tubercle.
Wound healing is inversely proportional to length.
The name of the prosthesis is based on the type of socket.

## PROSTHETIC PRESCRIPTION

Parts of transtibial prosthesis (Fig. 7.1) includes:

1. Socket
2. Suspension
3. Shin piece
4. Foot piece.

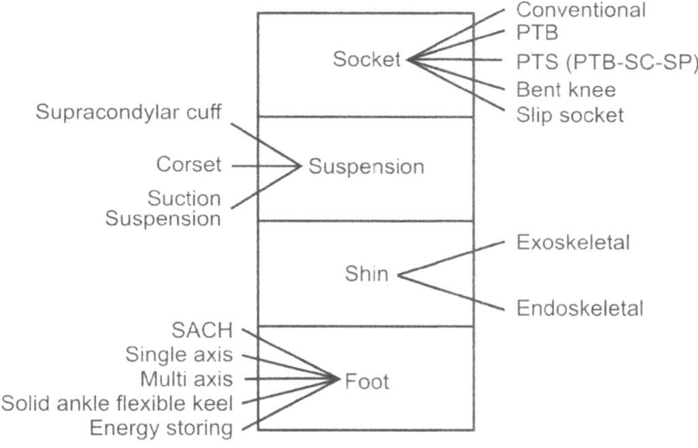


**Fig. 7.1:** A schematic representation of the parts of a transtibial prosthesis. The picture shows the most commonly used types of socket, suspension, shinpiece and foot assemblies used in India.

## 1. Socket

Socket is the part of prosthesis that encloses the stump and forms union between stump and artificial limb. Five types of socket are used. They are:

1. Conventional below knee socket
2. Patellar tendon bearing socket (PTB socket)
3. Patellar tendon bearing supracondylar suprapatellar socket (PTB-SC-SP socket)
4. Bent knee socket
5. Slip socket

### *Conventional Below Knee Socket*

These were the initial socket used in below knee before the PTB socket. It is indicated in elderly persons with unstable knee and persons with quadriceps weakness. It is fabricated in such a way that there is no pressure over distal tibia, head of fibula or tibial crest. 30% of weight by thigh corset.

It consist of a wooden socket, left open at the bottom. It requires external knee joint with thigh corset for stability and suspension. The major disadvantages are:

a. Skin irritation from friction
b. Stump chocking with edema over distal end of stump from constriction by the superior portion socket.

### *Patellar Tendon Bearing Socket (Fig. 7.2)*

Most commonly used socket in transtibial amputations. The socket is made of plastic over a mold of the stump and it is kept in 5 to 10 of knee flexion. 60% of weight is taken by patellar tendon and 40% by medial tibial flare. The anterior brim is at mid patellar level and lateral and medial brim and same level. The posterior rim is at popliteal crease.

The *pressure tolerant areas* are patellar tendon, medial tibial flare, lateral pretibial muscles, the popliteal fossa and gastrocnemius muscle.

The *pressure sensitive areas* are head of fibula, distal tibia, tibial crest distal end of fibula and hamstring muscles.

This type of socket can be fitted with supracondylar cuff suspension of external knee joint with thigh corset or suction suspension. It can be added with both exoskeletal and endoskeletal shin piece. All type of foot can be used. Soft insert can be provided if associated with sensory deficit.

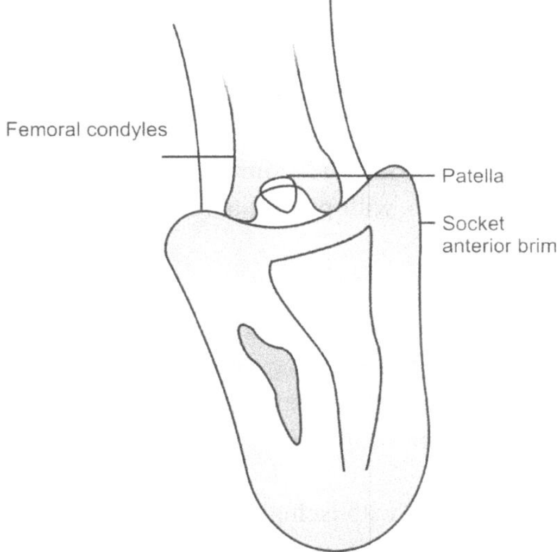


**Fig. 7.2:** PTB socket

### *Prostheses Tibial Supracondylien (Fig. 7.3)*

It is a French word and its equivalent is patellar tendon supracondylar and suprapatellar. The anterior trim line is supra patellar so that the whole of patella is inside socket. Same way lateral and medial trim line is supracondylar. This suprapatellar and supracondylar socket provides good suspension. So properly fabricated no suspension is required. It is useful in patient with short stump and patients with genu recurvatum.

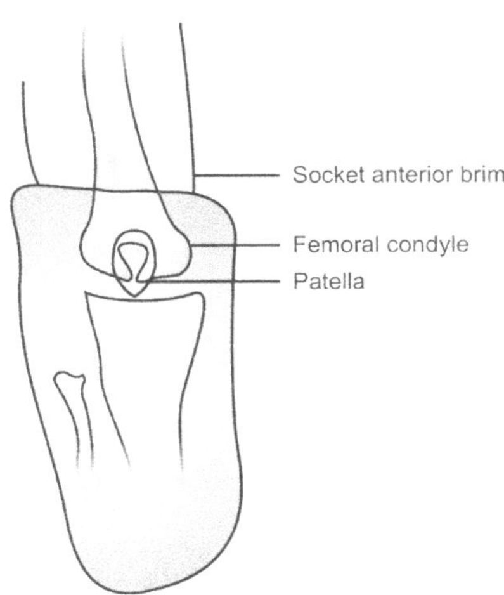


**Fig. 7.3:** PTS socket (PTB-SC-SP)

### *Slip Socket*

The socket is made of two layers – an external wooden or plastic socket and inner layer made of fine leather which fits to the stump. It is attached to the thigh corset by elastic layers. The outer layer pistons during swing. The prosthesis is fitted with external knee joint.

It is indicated in patients with painful adherent scar and in short stump.

### *Bent Knee Socket*

Indicated in conditions where fixed flexion deformity of stump cannot be corrected. Up to 20° of FFD can be accommodated in usual prosthesis. Flexed knee is a good position for prosthetic fitting. Weight bearing is based on clinical conditions of stump. Weight bearing may be:

a. Full end bearing
b. Proximal weight bearing with ischial seat
c. Partial at both sites.

## 2. Suspension

### *Supracondylar Cuff*

It is a simple cuff that suspends the prosthesis to supracondylar region around lower thigh closed by Velcro or buckle closure. This is the most commonly used suspension.

### *External Knee Joint with Thigh Corset (Fig. 7.4)*

It is indicated in patients with unstable knee, obese patients, aged persons and in short stump. It provides mediolateral stability as it is given with external knee joint with lock.

*Advantages:*

30 to 40% of weight is relieved by corset (through knee joint, prosthesis to ground).

*Disadvantages:*

1. Quadriceps wasting
2. Damages to clothes
3. Discomfort in hot weather
4. Non-cosmetic

### *Suction Suspension*

Silicone suction suspension—amputee rolls the suction socks over the stump and then attaches the socks to the socket with shuttle lock systems (Figs. 7.5A and B).

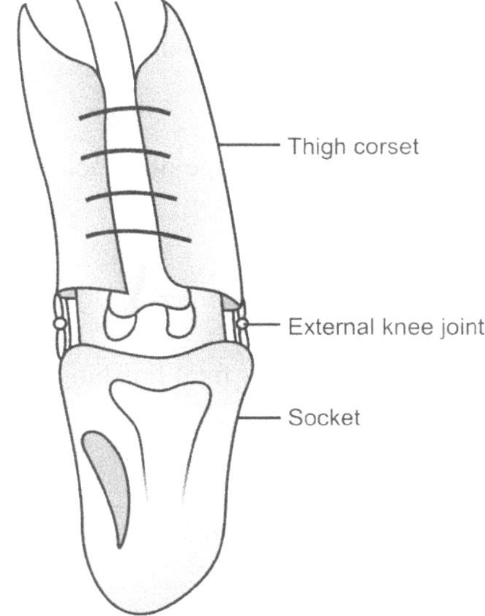


**Fig. 7.4:** Thigh corset

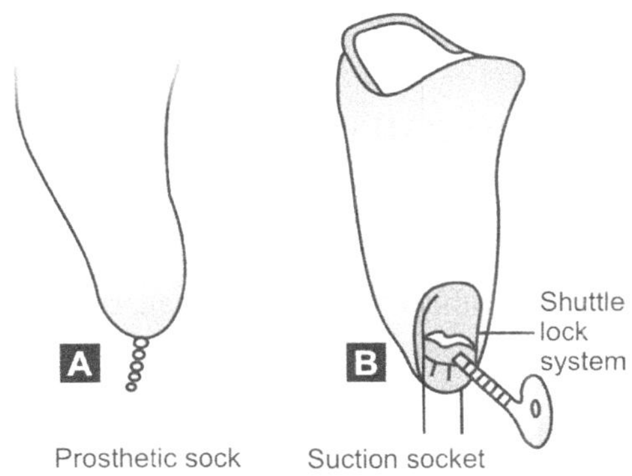


**Figs 7.5A and B:** Silicone suction suspension system. (A) Shows a silicone socks with a key at the lower end. Silicone socks rolled over the stump ensure a good skin-silicone interface. (B) Shows the shuttle lock system at the base of the socket. The key in the prosthetic socks is pulled through the lower end of the socket and is locked. This gives a good suspension for the prosthesis.

## 3. Shin Piece

*Exoskeletal (Crustacean)*

It is a hard outer plastic shell, moulded to the shape of leg.

*Advantages:*
Durable

*Disadvantages:*
Does not allow alignment change after finishing

### *Endoskeletal (Modular)*

This modular shin has a pylon to the shape of skeleton and a cosmetic foam cover to the shape of leg.

*Advantages:*
1. Lighter
2. Cosmetic
3. Adjustments can be done even after final finishing
4. Parts alone can be changed.

## 4. Ankle Foot Assembly

Five varieties of foot can be used in a transtibial prosthesis:
1. SACH foot
2. Single axis foot
3. Multi axis foot
4. Solid ankle flexible keel foot
5. Energy storing foot.

### *SACH Foot (Fig. 7.6)*

Solid ankle cushion heel (SACH) foot is the commonest foot used even in western countries. It is a foot with:

a. Solid heel made of wood or metal is directly attached to ankle block and there is no joint at ankle.
b. Cushion heel made of rubber heel wedge or alternating layers of soft and hard rubber. The compressibility of the cushion heel depends on patient weight and activity. This cushion heel compresses during heel strike simulating plantar flexion.
c. Molded cosmetic forefoot with or without individual toes.

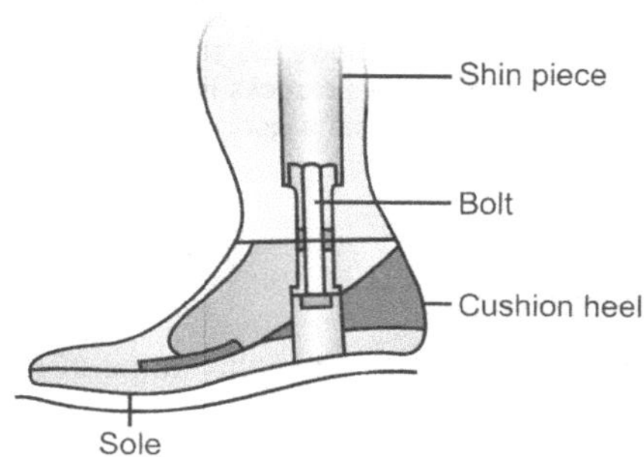


**Fig. 7.6:** SACH foot

*Advantages:*

1. Light weight
2. Durable
3. Little maintenance is needed
4. Near normal gait can be achieved.

*Modified SACH for Indian amputee are:*

a. Madras foot
b. Jaipur foot

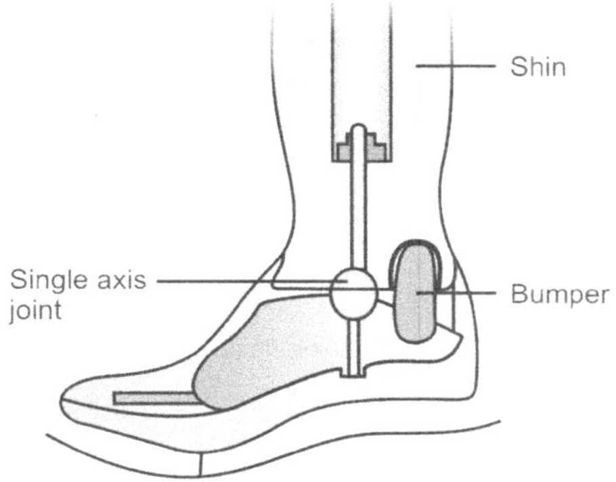


**Fig. 7.7:** Single axis foot

### *Single Axis Foot (Fig. 7.7)*

Allows limited plantar flexion and dorsiflexion by bumpers made of hard rubber. At heel contact plantar flexion bumper compresses causing plantar flexion and then foot flat. This rapid foot flat increases knee extension and causes prosthetic stability. So commonly used in above knee prosthesis.

### *Multi-axis Foot (Fig. 7.8)*

Allow dorsiflexion, plantar flexion, inversion and eversion and so provides good shock absorption. This foot is good for walking in uneven surfaces and excessively scarred stump.

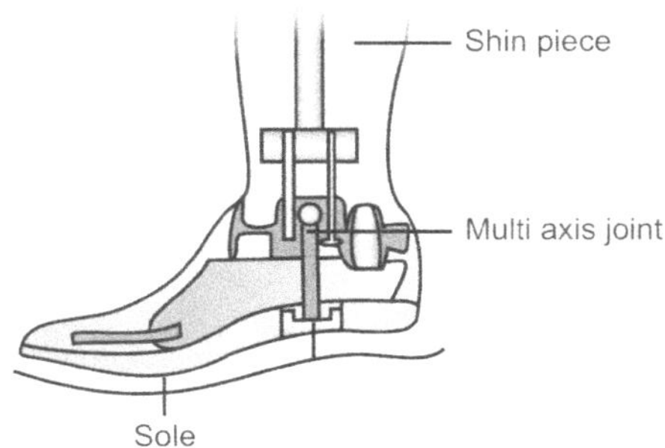


**Fig. 7.8:** Multi-axis foot

### *Solid Ankle Flexible Keel Foot (Fig. 7.9)*

Similar to SACH foot but with flexible keel. They offer better shock absorption and is useful in obese amputee.

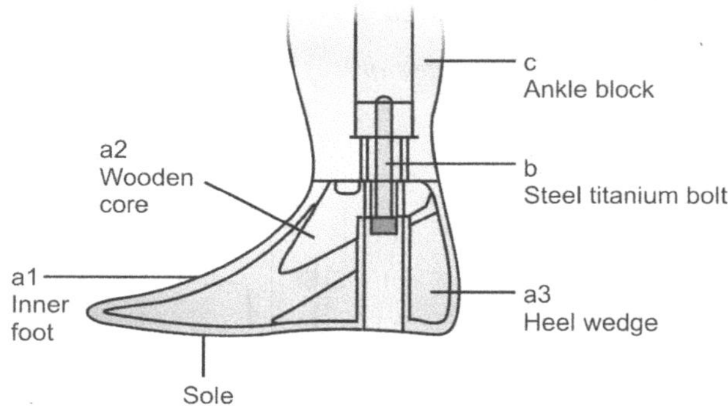


**Fig. 7.9:** Sold ankle flexible keel foot

### *Energy Storing Foot*

Also called as dynamic response foot developed initially for active and sports like running and jumping as. It consists of a shock absorbing leaf spring or carbon graphite that absorbs energy of heel contact and release it in terminal stance thereby providing propulsion. The patient can walk long time with energy foot than SACH foot. Energy efficient at high speed and is light weight. But it is expensive.

The prescription for prosthesis (Fig. 7.10) differs from person-to-person even if the level of amputation is same.

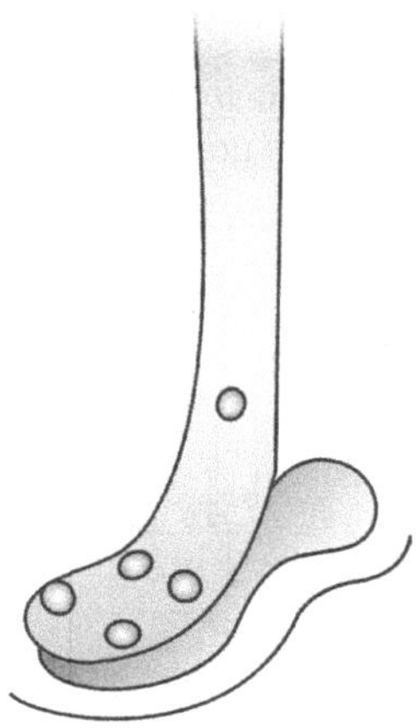

**Fig. 7.10:** Prescription of prosthesis

- *Prescription for good length stump:* Patellar tendon bearing total contact socket with supracondylar cuff suspension with exoskeletal shin with SACH foot with *boot* or madras foot with *chappal.*
- *Active young adult with sports activity:* Patellar tendon bearing total contact socket with **silicone suction suspension** with endoskeletal shin piece with **energy storing foot** with boot.
- *Aged with knee instability with diabetes:* Conventional below knee socket **with soft insert** with **external knee joint** with thigh corset with exoskeletal shin piece with SACH foot with *boot* or madras foot with *chappal* with back strap.

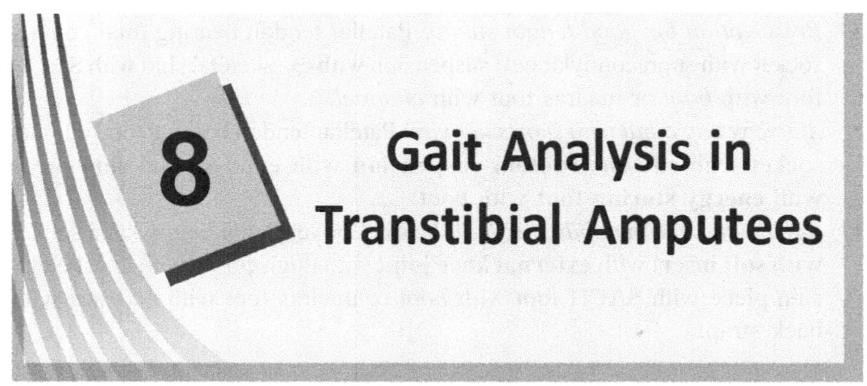

# 8 Gait Analysis in Transtibial Amputees

## BEFORE DONNING OF PROSTHESIS

1. Prosthesis meets specification and prescription
2. Inside of the socket is smoothly finished.
3. Joints if available are freely moving.

## SITTING WITH PROSTHESIS

1. Comfortable
2. Foot flat on ground
3. Adequate relief to hamstrings
4. Stump fit to socket
5. Suspension loosens/tightens.
6. Both knees at level
7. Color matching to normal limb.

## STANDING WITH PROSTHESIS

1. Interface between stump and socket (Too tight/too loose)
2. Knee stability and knee flexion
   a. Too much flexion needs leads to anterior knee pressure
   b. Too little flexion leads to end bearing.
3. Pelvis on level
4. Foot flat on standing
5. Gaping at brim of socket.

## WALKING

Check for:

a. Ball of foot more than 2.5 cm from floor
b. Knee extended on all phases
c. Unequal stride length.

## GAIT DEVIATIONS

### Heel Contact to Foot Flat

#### *Excessive Knee Extension*

In normal gait the knee flexes 10° to 15° on heel strike. It reduces movement of center of gravity and absorbs floor reaction force. Keeping knee extended increases energy expenditure and patient reports a sense of walking up hill. It also leads to distal pain and skin abrasions.

*Prosthetic causes:*

1. *Heel cushion too soft:* No rolling over possible and premature foot flat keeps knee in extension.
2. Posterior displacement of socket over the foot.
3. Excessive plantar flexed foot.

*Amputee causes:*

1. Weakness of quadriceps
2. Habit pattern.

- *Knee Instability*

1. Heel cushion too hard
2. Dorsi flexed foot
3. High heel shoe.

### Mid Stance

- *Excessive Raising of Hip*

Excessive raising of hip on prosthetic side is due to too long prosthesis.

- *Excessive Dropping of Hip*

Excessive dropping of hip on prosthetic side is due to:

1. Too short prosthesis
2. Painful stump.

#### *Wide Based Gait*

Support base is moved laterally so patient moves the pelvis and shoulders laterally exhibiting wide based gait. It leads pressure over proximal lateral aspect and distal medial area.

*Causes:*

1. *Out set foot:* Foot normally set 1 cm medial to a line from the center of posterior wall to floor. If foot is set too lateral to this line it is out set foot.
2. Medial leaning pylon or shank also leads to wide based gait.

*Narrow Based Gait*

1. Inset foot
2. Lateral leaning of pylon or shank.

## Terminal Stance

- *Drop Off*

The heel lever arm (back of heel to mid points if foot) provides support from heel strike to mid stance. Mid stance to terminal stance support is provided by to toe lever arm (mid point of foot to tip of toe) this helps the patient to roll over. Just before heel off knee is in extension and at heel off knee flexion begins. This change of extension to flexion coincides with passing of center of gravity over MTP joints. If the body weight is carried over too soon the lack of anterior support leads to premature knee flexion or drop off.

*Cause:* Toe lever arm too short.

- *Knee Extension Vaulting*

Too long toe lever arm causes extension moment at terminal stance (instead of the normal knee flexion moment at toe off). Patient complaints of walking up hill sensation as the center of gravity is carried up and overextended knee.

## Swing Phase

- *Pistoning*

The prosthesis slips as foot leaves the ground in swing phase.

*Causes:*

1. Loose or inadequate suspension
2. Loose socket.

- *Uneven Step Length*

Long step with prosthesis and short step with sound leg.

*Causes:*
1. Pain with poor fitting socket
2. Too long prosthesis
3. Fear of weight bearing.

- *Circumduction*

Semicircular swing of prosthesis during swing phase:
1. Too long prosthesis
2. Inadequate suspension
3. Flexor muscle weakness in hip and knee
4. Restricted flexion in hip and knee.

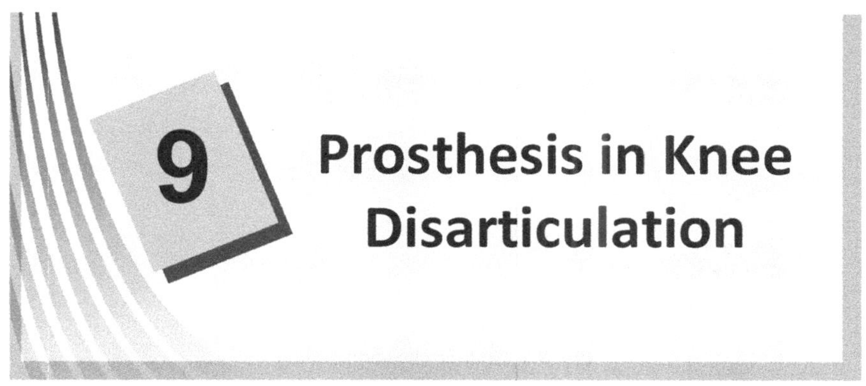

# 9 Prosthesis in Knee Disarticulation

## ADVANTAGES OF KNEE DISARTICULATION SURGERY

1. End bearing stump
2. Good rotational control
3. Good suspension
4. Less surgical time
5. Less blood loss.

## SURGICAL MODIFICATIONS

To improve cosmetic appearance of bulky condyles.

a. Limited trimming of condyles (Vauahen & Blank 1982)
b. Bone resection in medial, lateral, posterior condyles of femur and removal of patella (Mazet and Harmessey 1966).

Complications:

1. Reduction of weight bearing area
2. Oozing from raw cancellous bone, with a risk of hematoma
3. Infections
4. Necrosis.

## GRITTI-STOKES AMPUTATION (GRITTI 1857 AND STOKES 1870)

Resection the cancellous bone at the level of adductor tubercle and fusion of sliced patella to the distal condylar bone (Fig. 9.1).

## PROSTHESIS IN KNEE DISARTICULATION

Socket level depends on the weight bearing at distal end of the stump.

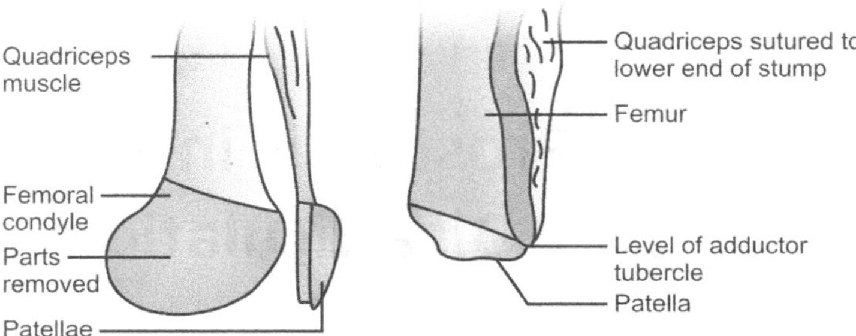


**Fig. 9.1:** Gritti-Strokes amputation

- **Socket**

a. *Full weight bearing by femoral condyles:* Femoral condyles bears weight and as well as provide suspension. The socket consist of a thin flexible brim that ends below ischium.
b. *Ischial weight bearing:* Quadrilateral socket with ischial weight bearing is given. A soft socket liner with supracondylar buildup provides suspension.

- **Knee Joint: Polycentric or external knee joint can be fitted**

Polycentric or external knee joint can be fitted. Polycentric knee joint is given to active young adults. External knee joint can be fitted with a lock in elderly patients and patients with hip extensor weakness.

- **Ship piece: Exoskeletal shank or endoskeletal shank can be given.**
- **Foot piece: SACH foot and single axis foot are used commonly. Atheletes and active young amputees are fitted with energy storing foot.**

## Deciding about Prescription of Below Knee Lower Limb Prosthesis

*Step 1:* Type of socket to be used

a. Stump length of 8 cm or more → PTB socket
b. Stump length of 3 cm - 8 cm → PTS socket
c. Stump length less than 3 cm → Bent knee or knee disarticulation
d. Fixed flexion deformity of more than 20 days → Bent knee
e. Aged patient/knee instability → Conventional below knee
f. Associated sensory deficit → Add soft inserts
g. Scarred stump → Slip socket or suction socket

*Step 2:* Suspension

a. Active adult → Supracondylor cuff (Cheap)
→ Suction suspension (Costly)

b. Unstable knee/ Overweight/Aged → External knee joint with thigh corset

*Step 3:* Shank

a. Durability → Exoskeletal
b. Cosmetic → Endoskeletal

*Step 4:* Foot piece

Decided based on the need of the patient.

| | *Advantage* | *Disadvantage* |
|---|---|---|
| a. SACH | – Light weight<br>– Durable<br>– Little maintenance<br>– Cheap | – Difficult in uneven surfaces |
| b. Single axis foot | – Quick foot flat improves knee stability<br>– Good shock absorption | – Heavier<br>– Less durable |
| c. Multi axis foot | – Good shock absorption<br>– Helps walking in uneven surfaces | – Heavier<br>– Less durable |
| d. Solid apple flexible keel | – Helpful in obese patients<br>– Good shock absorption | |
| e. Energy storing foot | – Very useful for active young adults, sports persons<br>– Good shock absorption | – Costly |

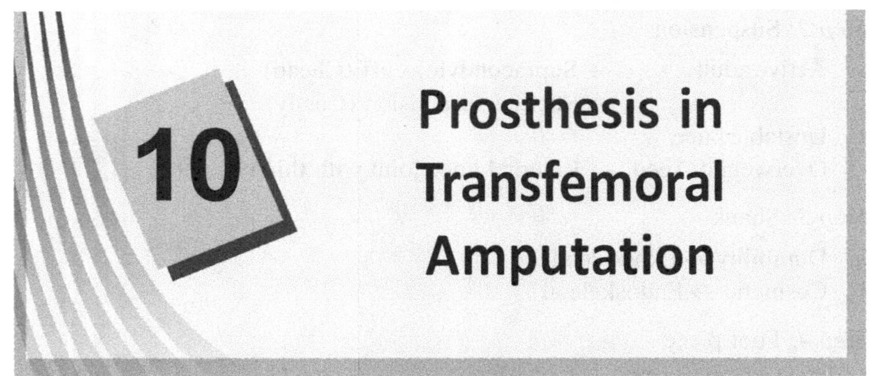

# 10 Prosthesis in Transfemoral Amputation

## PRINCIPLES OF TRANSFEMORAL AMPUTATION

1. Primary wound healing
2. Preserve as much length as possible
3. Maintain anatomical and mechanical alignment.

The mechanical axis of lower limb runs from center of head of femur through center of knee and to the mid point of ankle. The anatomical alignment, i.e. femoral shaft-axis is 9° from vertical. In most of transfemoral amputees, the stump is abducted due to over action of gluteus medius and minimus and loss of adductors at the level of insertion (expecially adductor magnus accounts for 70% adduction).

To prevent this complication, the adductors are sutured to the lateral aspect of femur with femur in maximum adduction. In addition quadriceps is sutured posteriorly and fascia lata is also sutured to femur.

## MUSCLE WASTING IN AMPUTEES

With the aid of MRI imaging with three-dimensional graphic reconstruction the amount of atrophy in muscles in stump after 2 years was assessed, it revealed.

a. Muscles that are not sectioned like gluteus medius and minimus, iliopsoas has 30% atrophy.
b. Muscles that lost insertion indirectly like gluteus maximus and tensor fascia lata due to non-attachment of fascia lata showed atrophy of 37 to 47%.
c. Muscles that are sectioned and attached by myoplasty or myodesis atrophied by 40 to 60%.

## TRANSFEMORAL PROSTHESIS

Difficulties encountered creating an effective prosthesis is due to (Fig. 10.1):

1. Weight bearing area (ischial tuberosity is proximal to propulsive structure) (thigh).

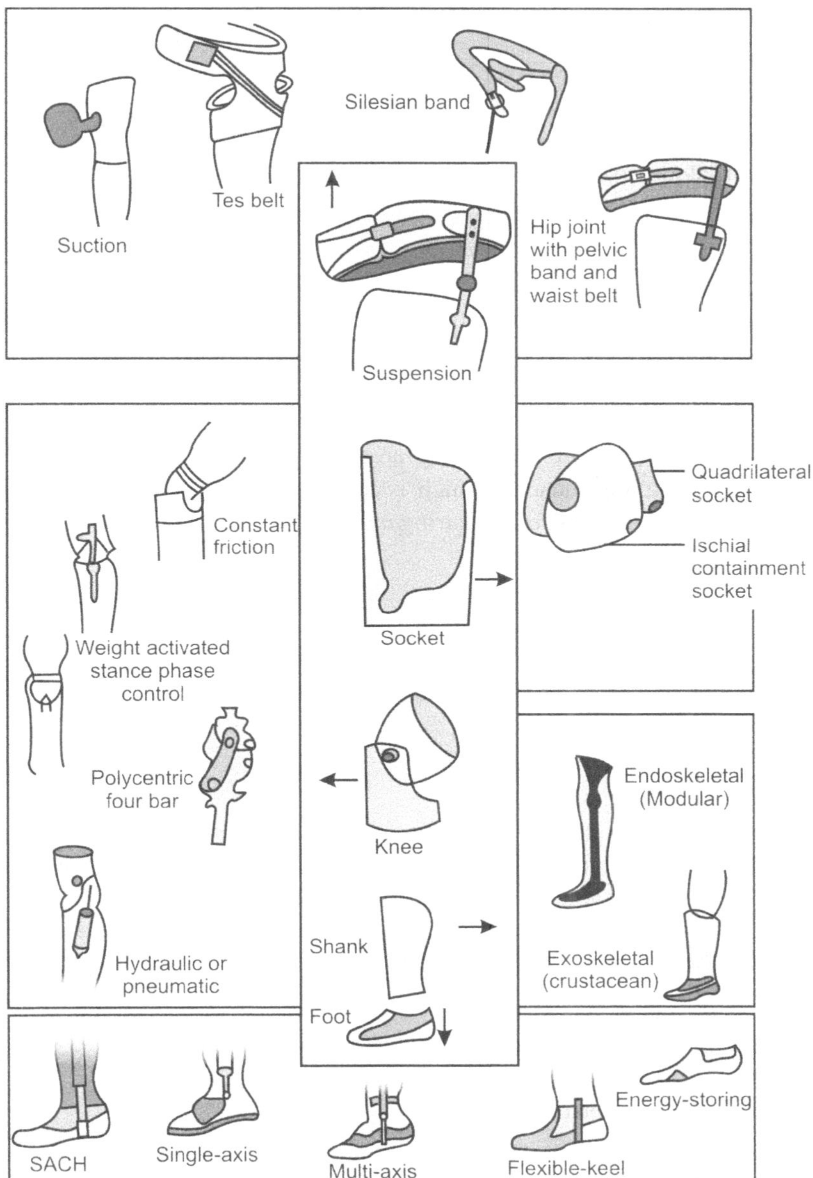


**Fig. 10.1:** Components of a transfemoral prosthesis–Common types of suspension, socket, knee joints, shank or skin piece and foot assembly used in India.

2. Passive mechanical replacement of 2 major joints (knee, ankle) and foot.
3. Limitations in prosthetic technology.

## • SOCKET

Two types of sockets commonly used are:
1. Quadrilateral socket
2. Ischial containment socket.

### Quadrilateral Socket

Developed late in 1950 and is named for its four walls. Distally the socket is contoured for total contact of residual limb.

#### *Posterior Wall*

It provides the major weight bearing area. It has an ischial seat for ischial tuberosity and glutei muscles which is thicker medially and thin laterally. Internally provides relief for hamstring muscle. Height of posterior wall is at the level of ischial tuberosity.

#### *Anterior Wall*

It extends five cm above the height of posterior wall with anteromedial inward femoral bulge called scrap's projection. It keeps the ischial tuberosity *in situ* anterior wall is convex laterally.

#### *Lateral Wall*

Normally, it extends, as high as anterior wall. For short stump it is in trimmed above trochanter to increase stability and control. The wall inclines medially with 10° adduction (normal adduction angle of femur).

#### *Medial Wall*

Medial wall is vertical and parallel to sagittal plane. Relief is given internally adductor longus anteromedially and hamstrings posteromedially.

### Ischial Containment Socket

Developed in early 1990 and shaped differently from quadrilateral socket. The ischium and a part of pubic ramus are enclosed in socket. It contains more area side socket so more area of weight distribution. Narrow mediolateral dimension helps in keeping up ischial tuberosity within posteromedial wall of socket.

The lateral wall covers trochanter to provide more stability. The distal socket is of total contact socket.

The two types of ischial containment sockets are:

1. CATCAM–Contour Adducted Trochanteric Controlled Alignment Method
2. NSNA–Normal Shape Normal Alignment.

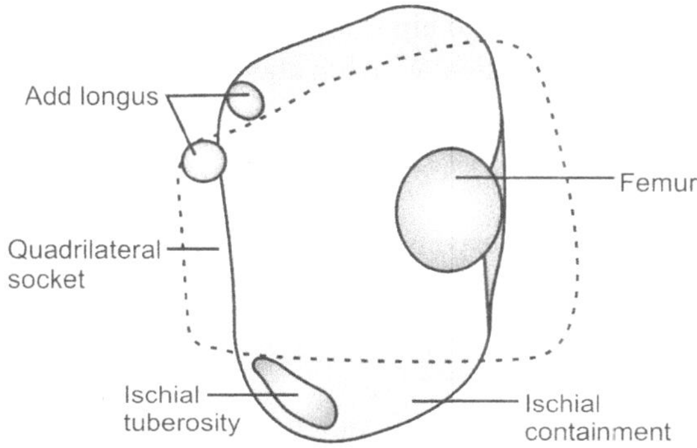


**Fig. 10.2:** Comparison of a quadrilateral and ischial containment socket. The dotted lines represent the quadrilateral socket wide in mediolateral dimension. The solid lines show the upper end of ischial containment socket with narrow mediolateral dimension with ischial tuberosity accomodated in posteromedial wall of the socket.

## Comparison Between Quadrilateral and Ischial Containment Sockets (Fig. 10.2)

| | *Quadrilateral socket* | *Ischial containment socket* |
|---|---|---|
| 1. | Quadrilateral with four walls | — |
| 2. | Ischial seat for weight bearing | No ischial seat |
| 3. | Femoral bulge present | No femoral bulge |
| 4. | Area of weight bearing is less | Area of weight bearing is more |
| 5. | Long lateromedial dimension | Narrow mediolateral dimension |
| 6. | Narrow anterioposterior dimension | Long anteroposterior dimension |
| 7. | Fair pelvic control | Good pelvic control |
| 8. | Fair rotational stability | Good rotational stability |
| 9. | Lateral wall normally extends below trochanter except in short stump | Extends above greater trochanter |
| 10. | Less energy efficient | More energy efficient |
| 11. | Indicated for standard stumps | It can also be used with short stump and gluteus medius weakness |

## • SUSPENSION

1. *Silesian band:* Commonly used. It is a leather belt fixed to the lateral side of socket. It encircles the body and attaches to anterior wall through buckles.
2. *Waist belt:* It provides more hip stability. It is with or without external hip joint. It can be used in patient with hip abductor weakness and short stump.
3. *Suction suspension:*
   a. Total suction
   b. Partial suction
   c. Hypobaric silicone suspension.

## • KNEE JOINT

1. Constant friction Knee Joint
It is a mechanical knee which provides knee stability during stance but no control during swing. It is a single axis knee allows flexion and extension. To prevent buckling patient should have good hip extensor. In case of weakness of hip extensor the axis of knee placed posterior to TKA line.

2. Polycentric Knee Joint
It allows flexion, extension and some rotation and it gives more knee stability. It is indicated in short stumps, aged patient and is hip extensor weakness.

3. Weight Activated Stance Control Knee
Also called as safety knee. The extent of friction depends on extent of weight bearing. The friction increases with increased weight bearing.

4. Hydraulic/Pneumatic Knee
They are cadence responsive through cadence dependant resistance. Initially these knee units were designed to provide control during swing phase only. Now they are modified to provide both swing and stance control.

a. Mauch S-N-S hydraulic knee where S-N-S is swing N Stance. It has a hydraulic cylinder and a swing adjustment with rod, thus providing swing control and resistance to knee flexion during stance.
b. *Endolite pneumatic intelligent prosthesis:* It has a computer controlled valve that adjust swing based on cadence.

## • SHANK PIECE

Both exoskeletal and endoskeletal shank can be used.

## • FOOT PIECE

Commonly used is SACH and single axis foot. Young active individual can be given energy storing feet.

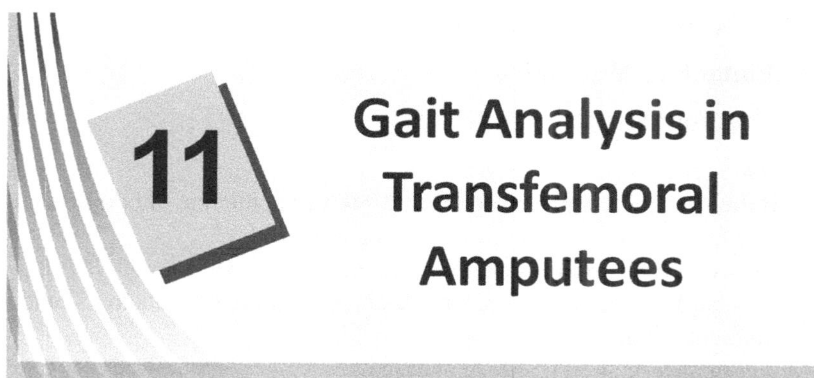

# 11 Gait Analysis in Transfemoral Amputees

Both static and dynamic evaluation has to be done.

## BEFORE DONNING OF PROSTHESIS

1. Prosthesis meet specification and prescription
2. Inside of the socket is smoothly finished
3. Joints moving freely.

## SITTING WITH PROSTHESIS

1. Socket is suspended securely
2. Shank equal to opposite side
3. Sitting comfortably without pinching
4. Able to learn forward to touch toes.

## STANDING WITH PROSTHESIS

1. Socket is fit properly
2. Knee is stable on weight bearing
3. Pelvis on level both sides
4. Socket is in good contact on all side
5. Adductor roll does not get pinched
6. Pressure on pubic ramus.

## WALKING

1. Heel rise adequate to clear ground
2. Prosthetic knee bends smoothly
3. Leg swings forward with adequate knee and hip flexion
4. Knee extends before next heel contact
5. Stride length equal on both sides.

## TRANSFEMORAL GAIT DEVIATIONS

### Heel Contact to Midstance

- *Knee Instability*

a. *Prosthetic causes:*
   1. If the knee joint is placed anterior to TKA line, the line of body weight will fall behind knee creating flexion moment.
   2. Inadequate flexion in socket limiting active hip extension.
   3. Too hard heel cushion less shock absorption also producing flexion moment at knee.

b. *Amputee causes:*
   1. Hip flexion contracture not accommodated in socket.
   2. Hip extensor weakness.

- *Terminal Impact*

Rapid forward movement of shank that leads to maximum knee extension before heel strike.

a. *Prosthetic causes:*
   1. Insufficient knee friction

b. *Amputee causes:*
   1. As habit by assuming to keep knee in full extension before heel strike.

- *Foot Slap*

Forefoot descends too rapidly like slapping the ground.

a. *Prosthetic*
   1. Plantar flexion resistance is too soft
   2. Heel lever arm is too short (end of prosthesis heel to mid point on foot)

b. *Amputee:*
   1. Forcibly driving foot into quick flat to assure extension of knee.

### Midstance

- *Lateral Trunk Bending*

All persons with transfemoral prosthesis exhibit some lateral bending from midline to prosthetic side. But excessive bending may be due to–

a. *Prosthetic causes:*
   1. Prosthesis too short causes hip drop as well as lateral bending
   2. Lateral wall is important for mediolateral stability. If lateral wall is fabricated with inadequate adduction angle it leads to lateral bending.
   3. High medial wall causing discomfort so lateral bending to avoid discomfort.

b. *Amputee causes:*
   1. Very short stump that fails to provide sufficient lever arm for pelvis.
   2. Painful stump
   3. Weak abductors in the prosthetic side
   4. As a habit pattern.

### *Abducted Gait*

a. *Prosthetic causes:*
   1. Too long prosthesis
   2. High medial wall pressure on pubic region so keep the prosthesis abducted.
   3. Improper fabrication and not maintaining adduction angle.
   4. Abduction contracture
   5. Pelvic band too far away from patients body.

b. *Amputee causes:*
   1. Abduction contracture
   2. Habit pattern.

- *Excessive Trunk Extension*

Hyperextend the trunk from heel strike to midstance.

a. *Prosthetic causes:*
   1. Insufficient socket flexion leads to lumbar hyperextension.

b. *Amputee causes:*
   1. Hip flexion contracture
   2. Weak hip extensors
   3. Habit pattern.

## Midstance to Heel Off

- *Drop Off*

Sudden downward movement of trunk as anterior support is lost prematurely.

a. *Prosthetic:*
   1. Socket placed too far anterior (toe lever arm short)
   2. Toe break placed posteriorly.

- *Inadequate Heel Off*

Heel may not come off floor till the whole body is brought forward.

a. *Prosthetic:* Uneven steps between two legs.

### *Circumduction Gait*

The prosthesis swings laterally like an arc during swing phase.

a. *Prosthetic causes:*
   1. Too long prosthesis
   2. Difficult knee flexion due to
      - Too much aligned knee (more posterior)
      - Too much friction in knee.

b. *Amputee causes:*
   1. Abduction contracture
   2. Not confident of flexing knee
   3. Fear of stubbing the toe.

### *Vaulting*

Patient rises on toe of the sound foot to swing the prosthesis through in the little knee flexion.

a. *Prosthetic causes:*
   1. Too long prosthesis
   2. Inadequate suspension
   3. Excessive knee friction
   4. Locked knee.

b. *Amputee causes:*
   1. Socket discomfort
   2. Fear of stubbing of toe
   3. Habit pattern.

### *Medial or Lateral Whip*

Medial whip is present when heel travels medially on initial flexion at the beginning of swing phase. Lateral whip exists when heel moves laterally.

a. *Prosthetic causes:*
   1. Lateral whip result from excessive internal rotation of prosthetic knee.
   2. Medial whip due to excessive external rotation of prosthetic knee.
   3. Too light socket
   4. Excess valgus, varus in the prosthetic knee.

b. *Amputee causes:*
   1. Applying prosthesis in internal or external rotation.

### • *Uneven Arm Swing*

Arm on prosthetic side held close to the body rather than freely swinging.

a. *Prosthetic causes:*
   1. Improperly fitted socket or unstable knee

b. *Amputee causes:*

1. Improper training
2. Fear
3. Habit pattern.

- *Uneven Timing*

Steps of unequal duration and length with short stance phase in prosthetic side.

a. *Prosthetic causes:*
   1. Improperly fitted socket causing discomfort
   2. Insufficient knee friction.

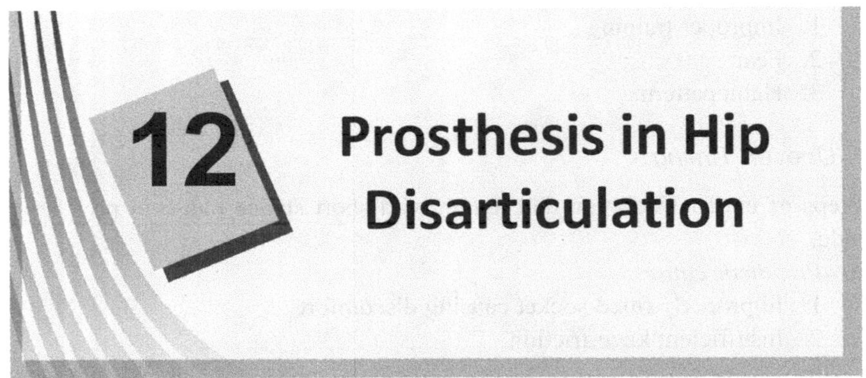

# 12 Prosthesis in Hip Disarticulation

Amputees with hip disarticulation can be fitted with:
Three types of prosthesis:

1. Tilting table type
2. Saucer type
3. Canadian type.

All types amputee bears weight through ischial tuberosity and gluteal muscles.

## TILTING TABLE TYPE

It is made of leather or plastic socket that encloses the stump and suspended by a pelvic belt and attached with external hip and knee joint.

## SAUCER TYPE

It is made of a very shallow saucer like socket over which the ischium, gluteal muscles sits. It has external hip and knee joints which can be locked. Because of shallow socket the stump tends to rotate and lessen the stability.

## CANADIAN TYPE

It is made of plastic or metal and it encloses ischial tuberosity for weight bearing and iliac crest for stability in swing phase. It has anterior/lateral opening for donning, doffing. Relief is provided for anterior superior iliac spine and posterior inferior iliac spine.

Mediolateral stability is provided by distal pressure on amputated side and proximal pressure over iliac crest on sound side.

Anteroposterior stability is achieved by position of hip and knee joint. Hip joint is placed on the anterior part of the socket and anterior to the direction of floor reaction force. The knee is placed posterior to the direction of floor reaction force. This keeps the knee extended (Fig. 12.1).

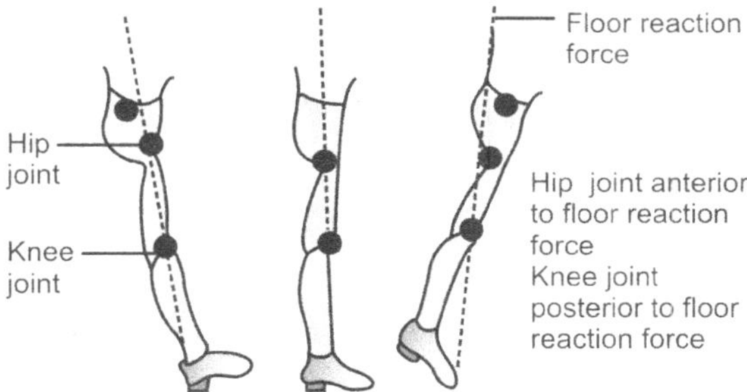


**Fig. 12.1:** Hip disarticulation prosthesis

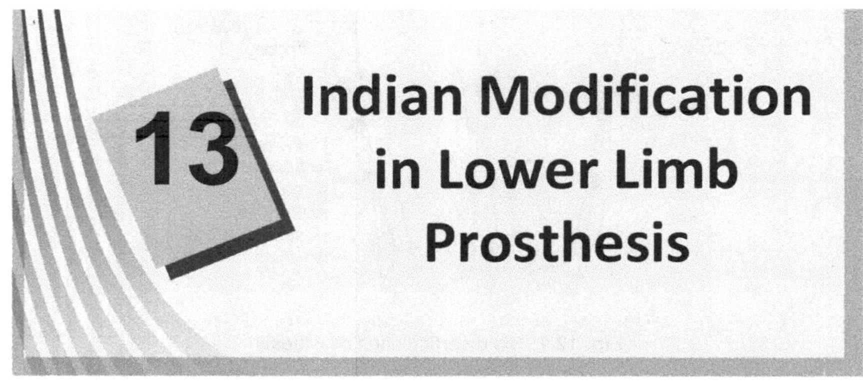

# 13 Indian Modification in Lower Limb Prosthesis

## Madras Foot

It is a modified SACH foot for bare foot walking. The modifications are:

1. The space between heel and ground is filled with sponge rubber
2. Toes are shaped like normal foot
3. Dorsum of foot is color matched and marked like normal foot
4. Tendo achilles like shape is made
5. Specialized rubber sole is made for bare foot walking.

## Jaipur Foot

It is also modified SACH foot with solid ankle and no ankle joint. The foot is made of galvanized rubber with shaping of toes. Instead of rubber polyurethane is used nowadays.

## Modification in Below Knee Prosthesis (PTB)

1. Posterior brim line is reduced and extends below popliteal crease to allow more knee flexion
2. The stability lost due to lowering brim line is compensated by raising lateral and medial brim line above condyles
3. The posterior portion of socket is made with flexible type of resin which yields on flexion
4. Elastic piece in supracondylar cuff to permit more flexion
5. A wedge shaped gap is provided at midtarsal level of foot piece to allow forward movement of shank over ankle.

## Modification in Above Knee Prosthesis

The thigh piece is divided into upper and lower. The lower piece rotates to 90° by turn table device to allow squatting.

# 14 Prosthesis for Hand Amputation and Wrist Disarticulation

## 1. TRANSPHALANGEAL

a. No device.
b. Cosmetic fingers or portion of a cosmetic glove.

## 2. TRANSMETACARPAL

a. Cosmetic glove
b. Open steel prosthesis shaped like an opposition semicircle
c. Mitt-shaped prosthesis

## 3. WRIST DISARTICULATION

### Disadvantages

a. On prosthetic fitting with wrist unit, the hand is longer than the normal side.
b. Close fitting prevents supination and pronation by 50%
c. Uncosmetic.

### Advantages

1. Myoelectric hand can be fitted.
2. If patient accepts, wrist unit with mechanical hand can be fitted.

### Prosthesis

1. Passive or cosmetic hand
2. Mechanical hand with Bowden cable operation for hand opening/closing
3. Myoelectric hand can be fitted.

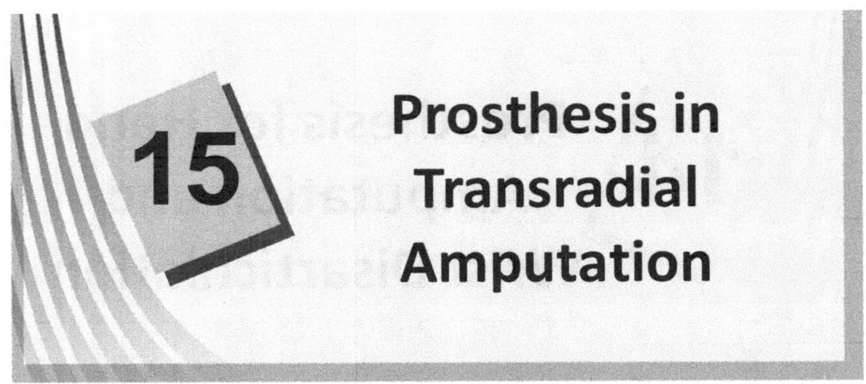

# 15 Prosthesis in Transradial Amputation

## LENGTH OF THE STUMP

First measure the length of normal hand from medial epicondyle to styloid process of ulna and that is taken as 100%. Then the stump is measured from medical epicondyle to lower end of ulna or radius which ever is longer in stump. Based on this, percentage of available stump can be calculated.

| | |
|---|---|
| 0-35% | Very short below elbow stump |
| 35-55% | Short below elbow stump |
| 55-90% | Medium below elbow stump |
| 80-90% | Long below elbow stump |

## TRANSRADIAL PROSTHESIS

A schematic representation of the parts of a transradial prosthesis has been shown in Figure 15.1. The types of suspension, cuffs, straps, elbow hinges, socket, wrist units, cable systems and terminal device available for transradial prosthesis are represented schematically.

## • SUSPENSION

### Figure of "8" Suspension

It consists of a loop around each shoulder. These loops are connected at the back and a 'O' ring may be placed at that place. One strap of the loop is connected to control cable and the other strap to inverted 'Y' suspension on the side of amputation. The loop on the sound side is called axillary loop (Fig. 15.2).

### Shoulder Saddle

It is indicated in person who do heavy manual work. (It has a large weight bearing area and no pull over sound axilla).

It suspends the prosthesis through bowden cable. The suspension cable attaches to 'Y' strap anteriorly and triceps pad posteriorly.

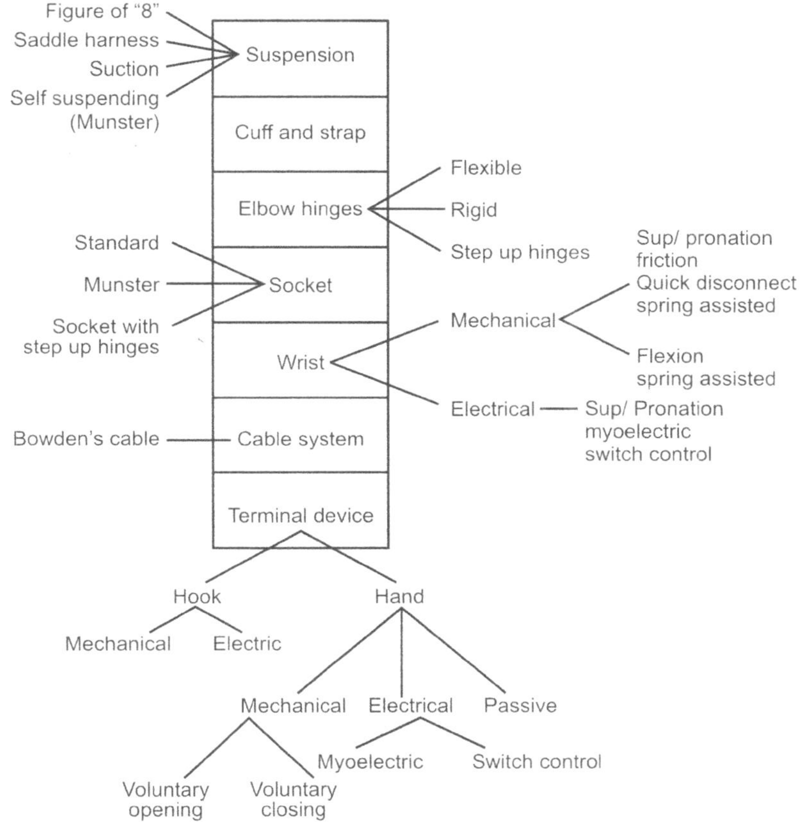


**Fig. 15.1:** Parts of B prosthesis

## Suction Suspension

Partial suction and hypobaric suction can be used.

## Self Suspending

In transradial munster socket design the bony prominences of humeral condyles are utilized for suspension. This suspension can be used in bilateral amputees and for patients with myoelectric arm.

## • CUFFS AND STRAPS

They are used to connect the socket with harness through elbow hinges. Triceps cuff is attached distally with elbow hinges and proximally with Bowden's cable and to figure of "8" suspension. Also by inverted "Y" suspension to figure of "8" suspension.

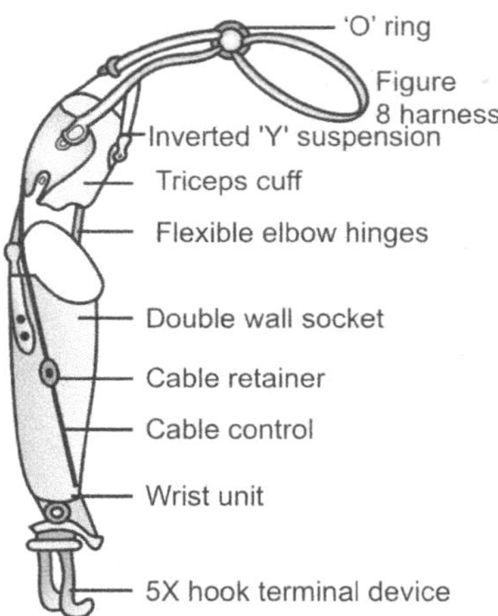


**Fig. 15.2:** A transradial prosthesis - with figure of '8' harness, O ring, inverted 'Y' suspension, with triceps cuff, with flexible elbow hinge, with double wall socket, with Bowden cable control with wrist unit of quick disconnect type with mechanical hooks—prescribed for a normal BE stump without complications.

## • ELBOW HINGES

They connect the socket to triceps cuff. The different types are:

### Flexible Hinge

This permits active pronation and supination. It is indicated is long below elbow and in wrist disarticulation.

### Rigid Hinge

For short BE stump with good flexion, extension at elbow. It provides stability of socket in all positions of elbow. It may be of single pivot, polycentric pivot, a multiple action and locking device.

### Step Up Hinges

Indicated in short stump with restricted range of movement at elbow. With this hinges one movement of stump leads to two degrees of movement of fore-arm shell of prosthesis.

## SOCKET

All the sockets are made of two walls. Inner wall corresponds to stump and outer corresponds to contour of the normal forearm.

### Standard Below Elbow Socket

With adequate length stump the upper rim located 1.5 cm below epicondyle of Humerus with elbow flexed at right angle. The trim line comes straight from ulnar side and curve distally to allow adequate relief for biceps muscle.

### Modified Munster Socket

Given to short stump with good range of movement at elbow. The trim line comes proximal to epicondyle with elbow slightly flexed and the posterior trim line goes above olecranon with elbow extended. It is self suspending and no additional suspension is required when properly fabricated. Extreme flexion and extension is restricted.

### Split Socket with Step Up Hinges

This is indicated in short stump with limited range of movement at elbow. With this arrangement with one degree movement at stump causes 2° movement at outer shell.

## • WRIST UNIT

Types of wrist units are mechanical and electrical units. Mechanical units are available pronation with supination and with wrist flexion. Commonly used are pronation, supination units which may be (a) Friction (b) Quick disconnect (c) Spring assisted. An externally powered switch or myoelectric control also available and not frequently used.

## • TERMINAL DEVICE

### Mechanical or Body Powered Hand

All functional hand uses three jaw chuck principle which involves grip with thumb index and middle fingers.

#### *Voluntary Opening Hook and Hand*

The hooks or fingers are kept closed by springs or rubber bands. It is opened by tension placed on control cable. Tension is provided by shoulder flexion in transradial amputation and by scapular abduction and chest expansion in above elbow amputations. Once the tension is released the hands closes automatically by springs or socket bands. This is preferred by most persons.

#### *Voluntary Closing Hand or Hook*

Kept open normally and needs tension to close the hand.

## Cosmetic or Passive Hand

Non functional hands constructed of semi rigid or rigid materials with cosmetic glove.

## Electrical or Externally Powered

Electrical or externally powered is of:

a. Myoelectric
b. Switch control

### *Myoelectric Arm*

EMG signals due to muscle contraction in the stump is utilized to operate externally powered prosthesis. It can be used to operate terminal device, wrist and elbow units. It may be of digital control i.e. on and off or proportional control is stronger signal gives a faster action. It consist of:

a. Electrodes
b. Amplifier
c. Battery
d. Motor

The electrical activity generated during muscle contraction is recorded by electrodes and it is amplified by amplifier and it is fed to the battery. The battery in turn operates the motor. The electrodes and battery are incorporated within socket or battery can be kept separately. Muscles in more distal portion of stump is to be selected. It should have normal innervations and voluntary control. Antagonistic muscles are used, i.e. elbow flexor or elbow extensor.

### *Single Channel Control*

Two electrodes one on the flexor aspect other on extensor aspect. Contraction of one muscle causes one action.

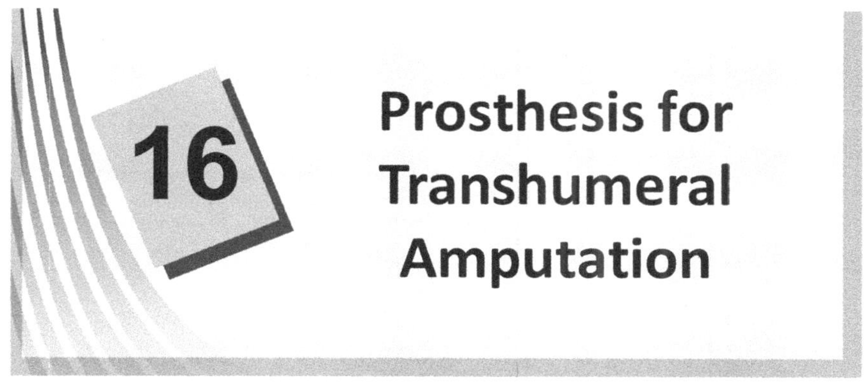

# 16 Prosthesis for Transhumeral Amputation

## Level of Amputation

Length of limb from acromion to lateral epicondyle on his sound side is taken as 100 percent.

Acromion to bony end on amputated side is calculated in percentage.

| | |
|---|---|
| 0-30% | Humeral neck |
| 30-50% | Short above elbow |
| 50-90% | Long above elbow |
| 90-100% | Elbow disarticulation |

Stump length of 7 cm can be fitted with a prosthesis (Figs. 16.1 and 16.2).

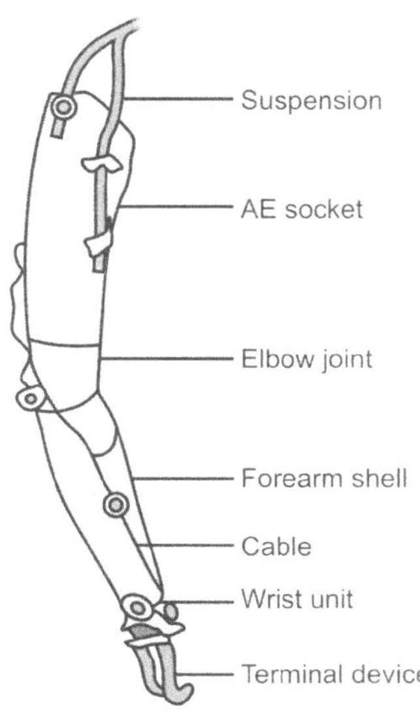


**Fig. 16.1:** Parts of a transhumeral prosthesis—supervision with figure of '8' harness with O ring with a Y strap, transhumeral socket $\bar{c}$ internal elbow joint $\bar{c}$ forearm sheel $\bar{c}$ wrist unit $\bar{c}$ terminal device with dual cable operating system.

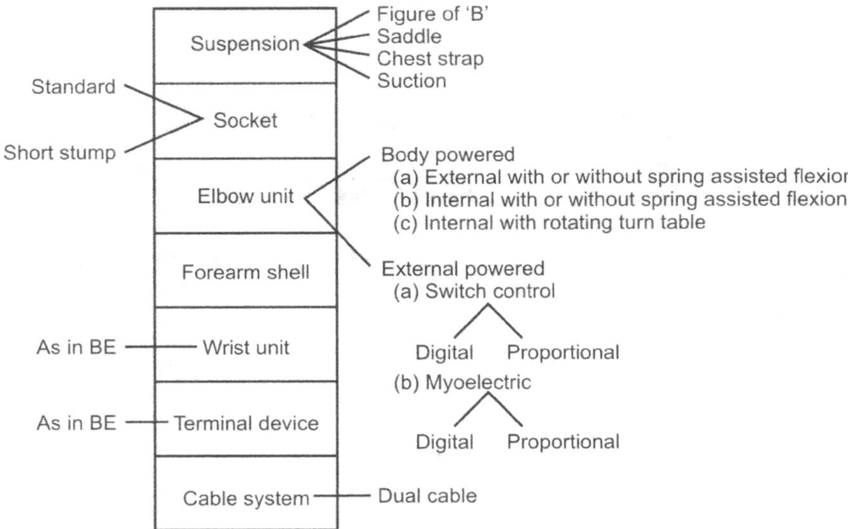


**Fig. 16.2:** Schematic representation of the types of suspension, socket, elbow unit, forearm shell, wrist unit, terminal device, cable system used in transradial prosthesis.

## Suspension

1. *Figure of "8" Suspension* has two loops in each shoulder which meets in upper back where "O" ring is attached. The anterior strap in Amputated side is directly attached to the socket. Posterior strap is attached to control cable.
2. *Saddle harness:* It suspends prosthesis though a cable which attaches anteriorly and posteriorly to the socket.
3. *Chest strap:* In humeral neck amputation, shoulder disarticulation and in forequarter amputations the chest strap is attached. It is attached to anterior and posterior aspect of socket.
4. *Suction:* As like below elbow, partial suction silicone suction suspension or hypobaric silicone suspension is used.

## Socket

Sandard Above Elbow Socket is used: For short AE (30-50%) and long (50-90%) AE slump. The trim line is 1 cm lateral to acromion.

## Elbow Units

*a) Body Powered:*

i) External with or without spring assisted flexion
ii) Internal with or without spring assisted flexion
iii) Internal with rotating turn table

b) External powered
   i) Switch control
      1. Digital
      2. Proportional
   ii) Myoelectric
      1. Digital
      2. Proportional

Internal elbow with rotating turn table allows limited rotation of forearm shell stimulating internal and external rotation of arm.

All body powered elbow operated by cable system. It is opened by shoulder depression, shoulder abduction and extension.

### *Forearm Shell*

Which is equal to the forearm that was present to which wrist unit is attached.

### *Wrist units – as discussed in Below Elbow Prosthesis*

### *Terminal device – as discussed in Below Elbow Prosthesis*

### *Cable System*

Dual cable system. One cable to operate terminal device by scapular abduction or chest expansion. The other cable to operate the elbow with shoulder depression and shoulder abduction or extension.

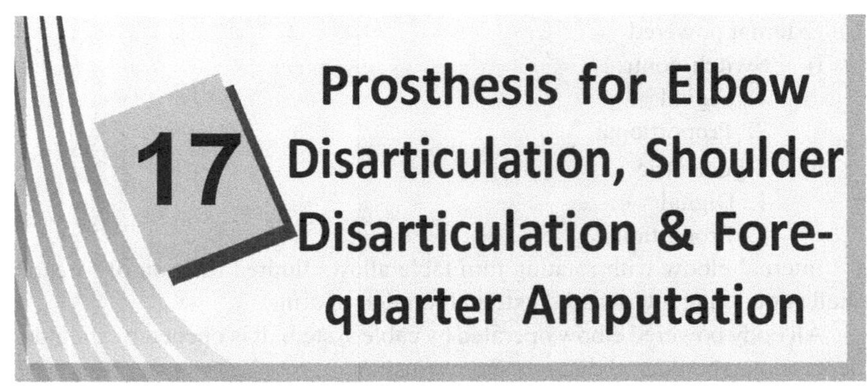

# 17 Prosthesis for Elbow Disarticulation, Shoulder Disarticulation & Forequarter Amputation

## Prosthesis for Elbow Disarticulation

Elbow disarticulation surgery is not commonly done.
*Advantages:* It can secure the prosthesis by its bony prominences
*Disadvantages:* It prevents rotation movement of forearm.

If internal elbow unit is used the joint level is 5 cm lower than normal side.

## Prosthetic Prescription

The prosthesis is made of double walled socket with rigid elbow hinges and external/internal elbow unit with forearm shell, wrist unit and terminal device.

## Prostheses for Shoulder Disarticulation

Shoulder disarticulation is usually done in patients with malignant bone tumors or electrocution.

Prosthetic prescription: The socket extends over a part of scapula and to rib cage anteriorly. Suspension is by means of shoulder strap. Elbow unit is similar to AE prosthesis. Cosmetic or functional terminal device can be provided.

## Prostheses for Forequarter Amputation

The socket covers a large area of rib cage anteriorly and posteriorly to provide stability and suspension by shoulder strap. Operating a functional terminal device is difficult at this level of amputation.

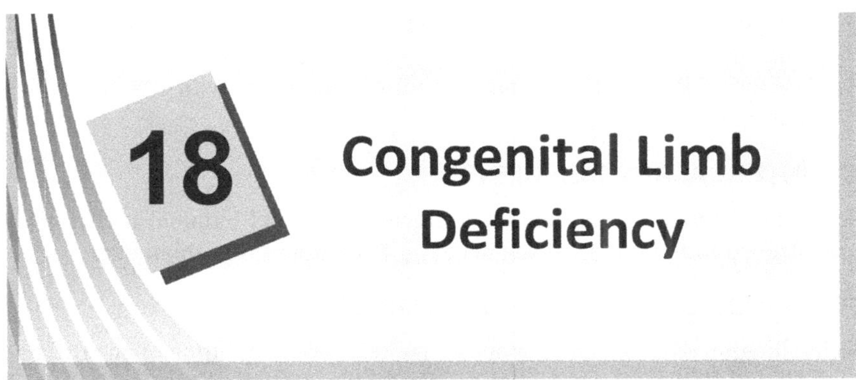

# 18 Congenital Limb Deficiency

Deficiency of absence of a limb at birth can be classified anatomically as follows:

## A. TRANSVERSE DEFICIENCY

It is defined as a limb that has developed normal, to a particular level beyond which no skeletal elements present. Buds may be present.

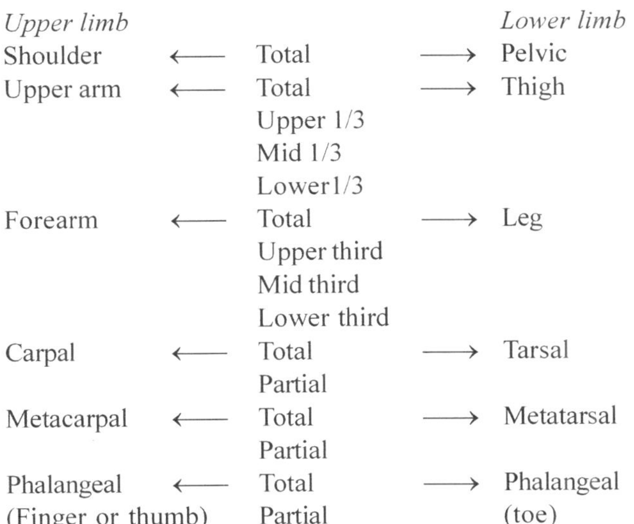

| *Upper limb* | | | | *Lower limb* |
|---|---|---|---|---|
| Shoulder | ⟵ | Total | ⟶ | Pelvic |
| Upper arm | ⟵ | Total | ⟶ | Thigh |
| | | Upper 1/3 | | |
| | | Mid 1/3 | | |
| | | Lower1/3 | | |
| Forearm | ⟵ | Total | ⟶ | Leg |
| | | Upper third | | |
| | | Mid third | | |
| | | Lower third | | |
| Carpal | ⟵ | Total | ⟶ | Tarsal |
| | | Partial | | |
| Metacarpal | ⟵ | Total | ⟶ | Metatarsal |
| | | Partial | | |
| Phalangeal | ⟵ | Total | ⟶ | Phalangeal |
| (Finger or thumb) | | Partial | | (toe) |

## B. LONGITUDINAL DEFICIENCY

Defined as a reduction or absence of an element or elements in the long axis of limb. It is named as per the following guidelines:

1. Name the bones affected in a proximal to distal sequence.
2. Affected bone is total or partially absence.

3. Number of digits should be stated in relation to metacarpal metatarsal and phalanges.
4. The term "Ray" refers to metacarpal or metatarsal with corresponding phalanges.

## C. INTERCALARY DEFICIENCY

Absence of forearm/arm/thigh/leg segment with intact terminal parts which are attached to the proximal segment e.g. Foot attached to thigh etc.

## PROSTHESIS IN CONGENITAL LIMB DEFICIENCY

Rehabilitation of a congenital amputee includes not only fitting of an artificial limb but also utilization of the residual limb as much as possible for functional independence.

### Upper Limb

Preservation of all available structures is recommended. Amputation of even deformed part to accommodate the socket should be done only after very careful functional evaluation as these children get trained easy to use the residual parts for the day to day activities (Fig. 18.1).

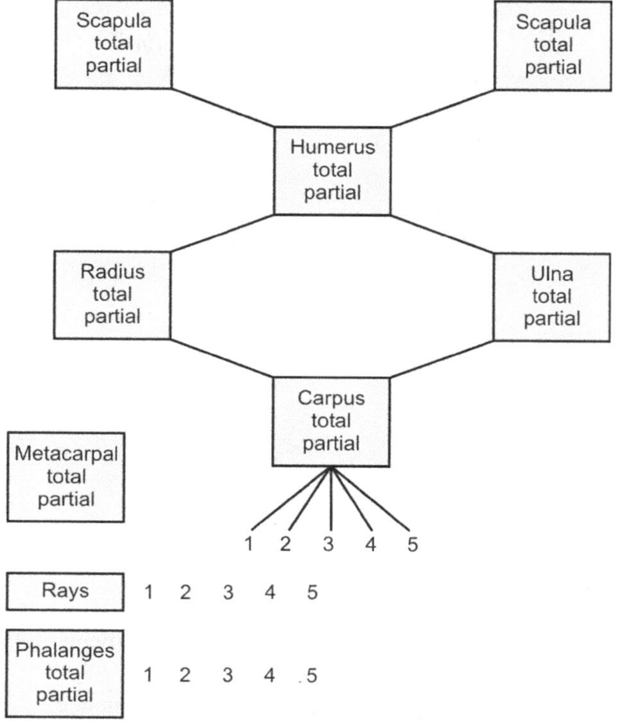


**Fig. 18.1:** Congenital transverse deficiency of upper limb

Prosthetic prescription is similar to any upper limb childhood amputee with custom made sockets to accommodate the available stump. First prosthesis is recommended around one year of age when a normal child learns bimanual activities.

Choice of terminal device and control systems need to be reviewed as the child grows to match their needs.

## Lower Limb

Prosthetic fitting in lower limb is mainly decided based upon the following criteria like weight bearing area, deformity in bones which will after the line of weight bearing, joints available and their functions, limb length discrepancy, etc (Fig. 18.2).

Surgical correction of residual limb for prosthetic fitting is usually done in lower limb congenital deficiencies. But in case of multiple deficiencies including upper limb deficiency, functional adaptations of foot (even if deformed) is considered before decision of amputation is taken.

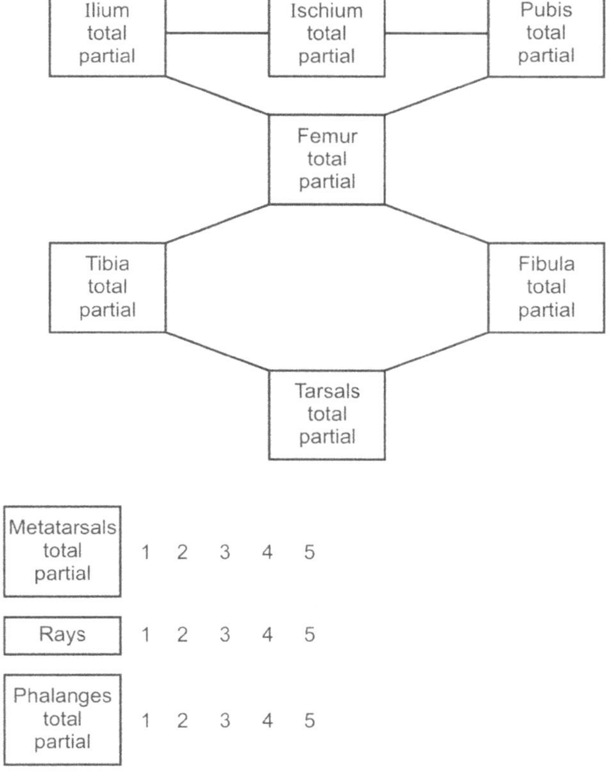


**Fig. 18.2:** Congenital transverse deficiency of lower limb

Most commonly prescription of a lower limb congenital amputee (intercalary or transverse deficiency) is

a. Extension type of prosthesis with socket with ischial/PTB weight bearing or with a foot plate for weight bearing. Joints and foot piece are like any other amputee.
b. Extension type of orthosis with ischial seat or foot plate for weight bearing. Most commonly it is a HKAFO/KAFO modified to meet the needs of the patient.
c. Shoe lifts

In case of longitudinal deficiencies, patients are fitted with supportive orthosis to ensure proper transmission of weight like HKAFO/KAFO/AFO etc. If the limb is not able to bear weight, amputations are considered to ensure proper or better gait.

Children with lower limb deficiencies are to be fitted with prosthesis at age of 6 months to aid proper sitting balance. Upto the age of 4 years no joint is fitted in the prosthesis.

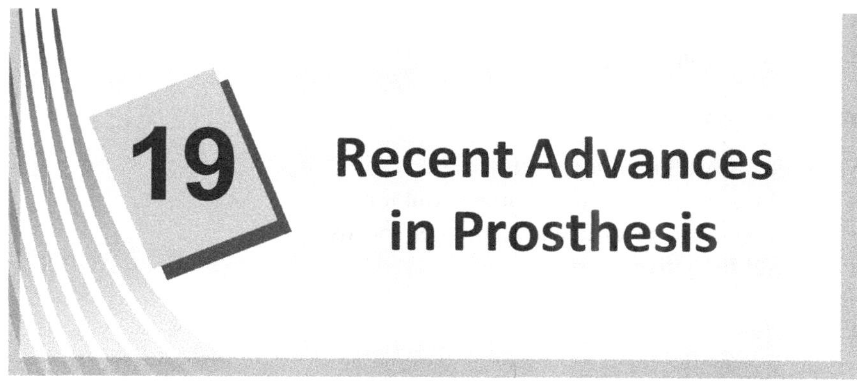

# 19 Recent Advances in Prosthesis

Development in all fields of technology reflects in advancement of prosthetic components.

## • SOCKET

Two models of ischial containment socket in transfemoral prostheses
1. CATCAM: Contour adducted trochanteric controlled alignment method.
2. NSNA: Normal shape normal alignment

## • SUCTION SUSPENSION

a. Total suction suspension. Steps in using suction suspension is as follows:
   - Pull socks over the stump
   - Insert the stump in the socket and pull the socks
   - One way valve closes the socket.

b. Partial suction
   - Prosthetic socks is pulled over the stump
   - Socket has a suction valve
   - Suction valve + prosthetic socks gives partial suction only
   - Auxiliary suspension is required.

c. Hypobaric silicone suspension
   - Gives better suction in loose fitting socket.

## • ENDOSKELETAL SHANK

- Lighter is weight
- Cosmetic
- Adjustment even after final finishing
- Parts can be changed.

## • ENERGY STORING FEET (DYNAMIC RESPONSE FEET)

- Stores energy when weighted and release energy when unweighted

- Gives a springy feeling
- Made of graphite springs.

## Advantages

- Speed of walking increased
- Slight energy efficient in normal walking
- Increased energy efficiency at higher speeds
- Useful for active sports.

*Examples*

- Carbon copy II, Light
- Carbon copy III
- Flex walk
- Spring lite.

## • CAD/CAM (COMPUTER AIDED DESIGN/ COMPUTER ASSISTED MANUFACTURING)

- MRI image
- Ultrasound image
- Video image

(MRI, ultrasound and video images: All are fed to the computer)

- Computer controlled carver makes the positive mould.
- Socket can be fabricated from it.

## "C" LEG

- Microprocessor controlled prosthesis.
- Knee/shin systems with hydraulic swing/stance control.
- In above knee prosthesis
- Used commonly.

## • TERMINAL DEVICE AND ELBOW MECHANISM

A. *Electric switch control mechanism:* Switch operated by residual limb movement

B. *Myoelectric control:*
   - Electrical activity generated during muscle contraction to control the flow of energy from battery.
   - Antagonistic muscles are used:
     - One for hand closure
     - Other for hand opening.

C. Verbal command control
   - Operate on verbal commands.

# Section II

# ORTHOSIS

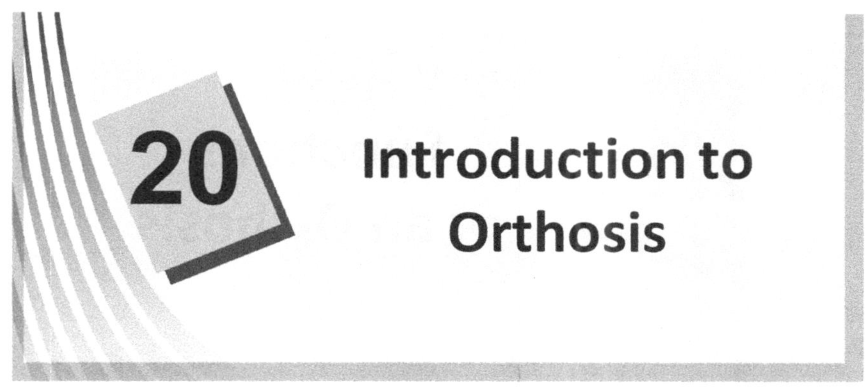

# 20 Introduction to Orthosis

## DEFINITION

An orthosis is defined as an externally applied device used to modify structural and functional characteristics of neuromusculoskeletal system.

Orthosis is a Greek word meaning "making straight".

Confusing different terminology used to describe it as braces, splints, calipers, appliances. In 1972 new terminology was developed and put into use. It is described by:

a. Joint it encompasses
b. Abbreviating each joint into single letter
c. By using combination of symbols to describe the orthosis
d. Add up "O" refers to orthosis at the end.

### Example

KAFO—Knee ankle foot orthosis
TLSO—Thoracolumbar sacral orthosis.

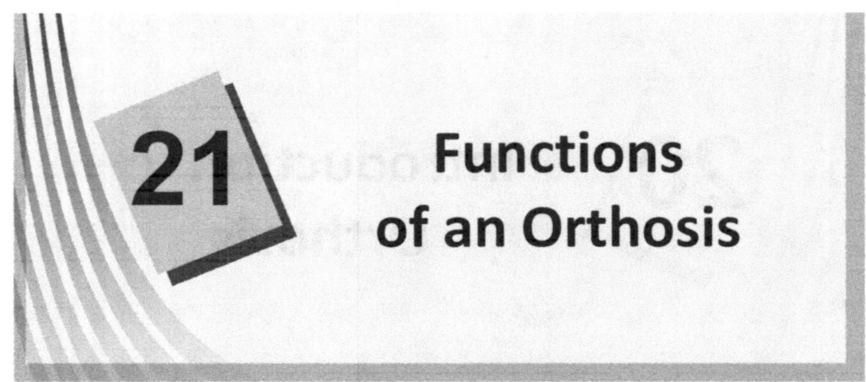

# 21 Functions of an Orthosis

1. To assist weak part or segment, e.g. springs, rubber bands, flexor hinge hand orthosis.
2. To resist movement at a joint or part, e.g. foot drop stop to resist plantar flexion.
3. *To support:* To give rest or immobilize a joint or part to allow heal up, to prevent deformity or to maintain is functional position.
4. *To substitute for absent motor function:* The patient moves hand in one direction and when relaxed the orthosis moves the segment in opposite direction, e.g. dynamic finger extension split in radial nerve injury.
5. *To relieve weight:* Weight relieving orthosis, e.g. ischial or PTB weight relieving orthosis.
6. Attachment of Assistive devices, e.g. universal cuff to which assistive devices can be attached.
7. To block a particular segment to prohibit movement in one joint so that the other joints can be exercised, e.g. orthosis with finger MP stop to allow movements in IP joints. This allows strengthening of flexor digitorum sublimis, e.g. knuckle bender splint in claw hand.

Orthosis can be made of metal moldable plastic, polyurethane foam, rubber, epoxy resin or plaster of Paris. Orthosis may be:

1. Static
2. Dynamic.

## STATIC ORTHOSIS

It is an orthosis that is rigid and gives support without any movement.

1. Support the segment in functional position preventing stiffness and contracture.
2. Also used to correct deformity by serial splinting.

## DYNAMIC ORTHOSIS

It is used to keep limb in position and allows movement in specific directions.

1. Support the segment of extremity.
2. Preventing stiffness of joint.
3. Strengthen and re-educate the muscle.
4. Mobilize the joint in desired position.
5. Assist in activities of daily living.

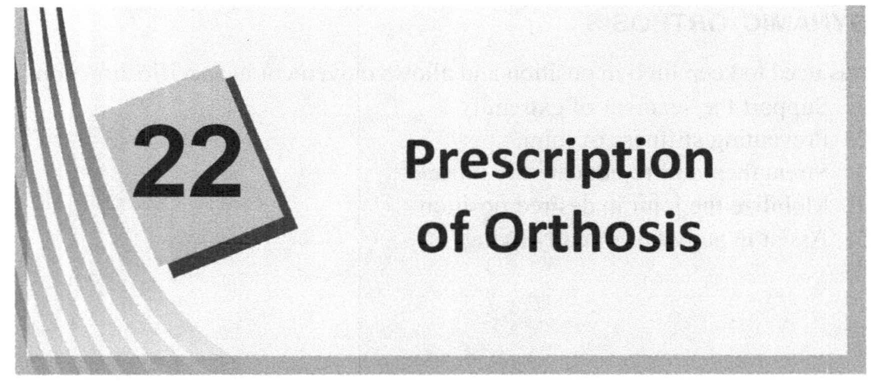

# 22 Prescription of Orthosis

Orthoses are given to the following conditions:

1. Post polio paralysis
2. Nerve injuries
3. Stroke and trauma brain injury
4. Spinal cord injury
5. Arthritis and soft tissue rheumatism
6. Deformities
7. Congenital limb deficiency
8. Burns
9. Sports.

Before prescribing as orthosis the following points are to be considered.

1. Range of motion in joints
2. Muscle strength
3. Sensation
4. Spasticity
5. Deformities
6. Shortening
7. Pain
8. Vocational, avocational needs
9. Durability
10. Utility
11. Simplicity
12. Comfortability
13. Cosmeticity.

Orthosis used in different regions is described separately. They are:

1. Spinal orthosis
2. Upper limb orthosis
3. Lower limb orthosis
4. Foot wear modifications

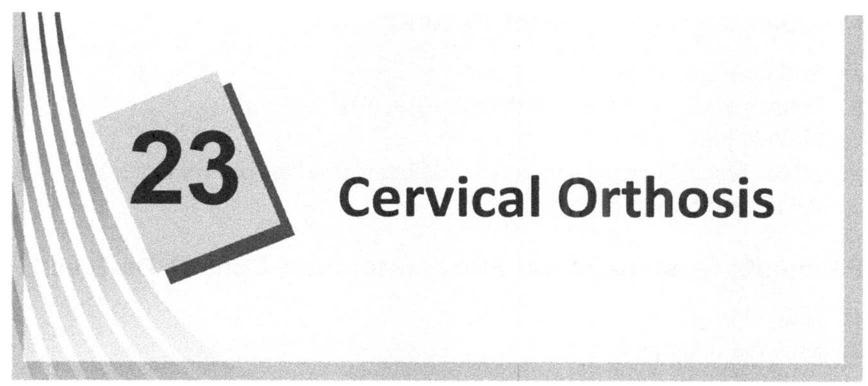

# 23 Cervical Orthosis

Cervical orthosis includes devices used in treatment of disorders around the region of neck and skull.

Immobilizing cervical spine is difficult because:
a. Most mobile part in spine
b. Has small body surface
c. Limited pressure tolerant areas like chin, occiput
d. Different types of predominant movement at different levels.

## FUNCTIONS OF CERVICAL ORTHOSIS

1. Positions the head
2. Limits movement in flexion, extension, rotation and lateral rotation
3. Unload the cervical spine by bearing part of weight of skull.

### Classification

Cervical orthosis can be classified as:
1. Cervical collars
2. Poster appliances
3. Cervicothoracic orthosis
4. Halo devices.

Commonly used are:
a. Soft and semi rigid cervical collars
b. Philadelphia orthosis
c. SOMI brace
d. Poster orthosis
e. Yale type of cervicothoracic orthosis
f. Minerva body jacket
g. Halo jacket or vest.

## Flexion/Extension Control Devices

a. Soft cervical collar
b. Semirigid cervical collar with chin—Occiput support
c. Philadelphia orthosis
d. SOMI brace (Sterno Occiputo Mandibular Immobilization Brace)
e. Poster orthosis

## Flexion/Extension/Lateral Flexion/Rotation Control Devices:

1. Halo vest
2. Minerva body jacket.

- *Cervical Collars*

### *a. Soft cervical collar*

It is made of foam and rubber covered by a stockinet.

*Advantages:*
1. Low cost
2. Easy to fabricate
3. Tolerated by patient
4. Provides warmth and psychological comfort.

*Disadvantage:* Does not restrict cervical motion in any plane and serves only as a remainder to hold neck and avoid excessive movement.

### *b. Semi-rigid Cervical Collar*

It is made of rigid polypropylene. Height of the orthosis can be changed by adjusting the two parts of collar.

*Advantages:*
1. Easy to apply and remove
2. Some restriction of flexion and extension
3. Chin and occipital extension can be added.

*Disadvantage:*
a. Does not restrict lateral bending and rotation.
b. Can press on clavicle and give discomfort.

- *Philadelphia Orthosis*

Philadelphia orthosis is made of plastozole reinforced with anterior and posterior struts. It has molded mandibular and occipital support. Anteriorly and posteriorly it extends to upper thorax (Fig. 23.1).

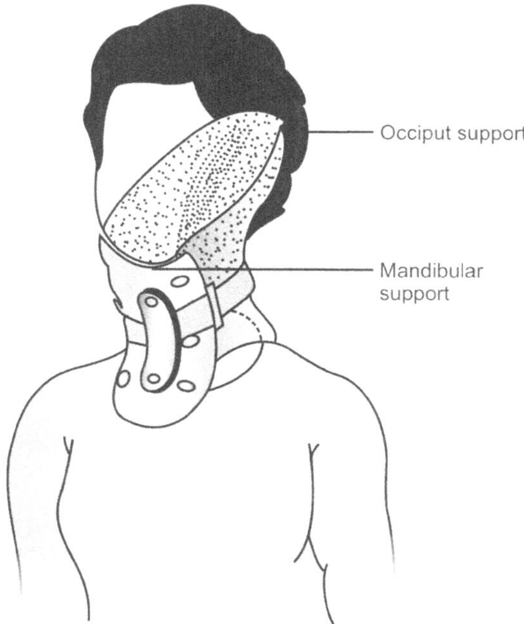


**Fig. 23.1:** Philadelphia collar: A semirigid cervical orthosis with mandibular and occiput supports and anterior, posterior struts. Restricts flexion, extension of cervical spine.

*Advantages:*

1. Restricts flexion extension due to chin and occiput support and thoracic extension.

*Disadvantage:*

a. Ineffective in controlling rotation and lateral bending
b. Pressure over clavicle.

- *SOMI Brace*

Sterno Occipito Mandibular Immobilization brace. It is a modified poster appliance. It consists of a sternal plate (Fig. 23.2).

a. One anterior strip which hold chin support
b. Two rigid metal rods from anterior to posterior to occiput support.

*Advantages:*

1. There is no posterior post. So it can be used with patient lying supine.
2. Light weight donning and doffing.

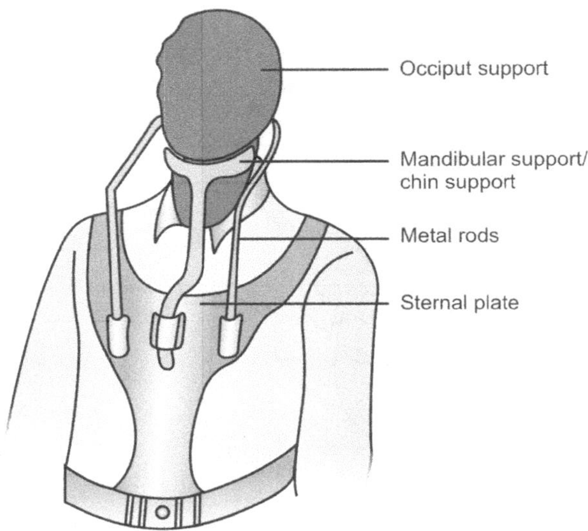


**Fig. 23.2:** SOMI Brace: Sterno occiputo mandibular immobilisation brace–A modified poster appliance with chin, occiput support and 2 metal rods from anterior to posterior and a sternal plate. There is no posterior post.

- *Poster Appliances*

It has anterior section consisting of sternal support, one or two uprights and chin support. Posterior section consist of thoracic plate, one or two uprights and an occipital support.

It limits flexion, extension, rotation and lateral flexion. It also unloads the cervical spine by chin and occiput support. Two varieties are (Fig. 23.3):

1. Four poster orthosis (Thomas collar)
2. Two poster orthosis (Peter Cervicothoracic orthosis) which provides less lateral stability.

- *Yale Cervicothoracic Orthosis*

Yale cervicothoracic orthosis is a modified philadelphia collar with plastozole reinforced with struts.

It extends down to mid thorax anteriorly and posteriorly. Occipital support extends higher on skull. With extended area of support stability is increased.

- *Halo Device*

Halo devices are used for treating cervical fractures and dislocation. It consist of:

a. Rigid metal or graphite ring attached to skull by four fixation pins
b. Four posters which are attached to ring proximally-two anteriorly, two posteriorly and distally to polypropylene vest.

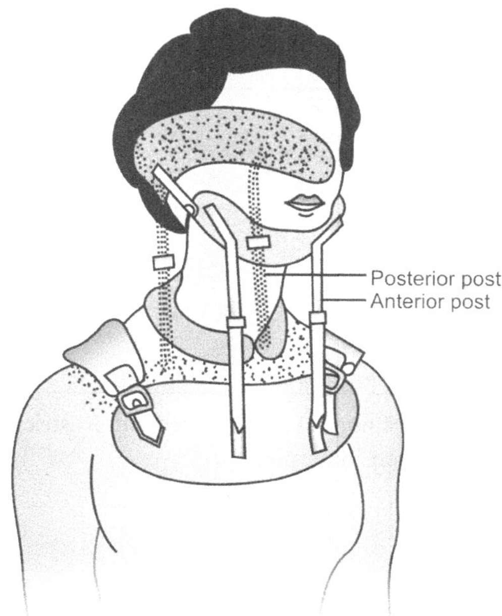


**Fig. 23.3:** Four Poster Orthosis - Thomas collar - Has 2 anterior posts and 2 posterior posts - Limits flexion, extension, rotation and lateral flexion. Also unloads the cervical spine by chin and occiput support.

c. *Polyethylene vest:* The vest may be of:
   i. Half vest—Level of nipples for upper cervical injuries
   ii. Short extended vest up to the level of 12th rib
   iii. Full vest—Level of iliac crest for lower cervical injuries.

- *Minerva Body Jacket*

This is an orthosis made of Plaster of Paris or Thermo Plastic

It consist of:

a. Forehead adaptation with occipital support
b. Chin support
c. Body jacket that extends up to the level of twelfth rib or umbilicus.

*Advantages:*

1. Light weight (plastic)
2. No invasive pins like halo device

It limits flexion, extension, rotation and lateral rotation like halo. Halo device and Minerva body jacket are the choice in ambulant management of unstable cervical spine.

## NORMAL MOTION VS RESTRICTION OF NECK MOVEMENT WITH ORTHOSIS

| *No.* | *Names of orthosis* | *Flexion extension* | *Lateral bending* | *Rotation* |
|---|---|---|---|---|
| 1. | Normal | 100 | 100 | 100 |
| 2. | Soft collar | 25 | 8 | 16 |
| 3. | Philadelphia | 71 | 33 | 56 |
| 4. | SOMI | 72 | 34 | 64 |
| 5. | Four poster | 80 | 54 | 82 |
| 6. | Halo | 89 | 92 | 98 |
| 7. | Minerva body jacket | 77 | 76 | 100 |

100 is the percentage of normal neck movement. Restriction of movement offered by orthoses is given in percentage.

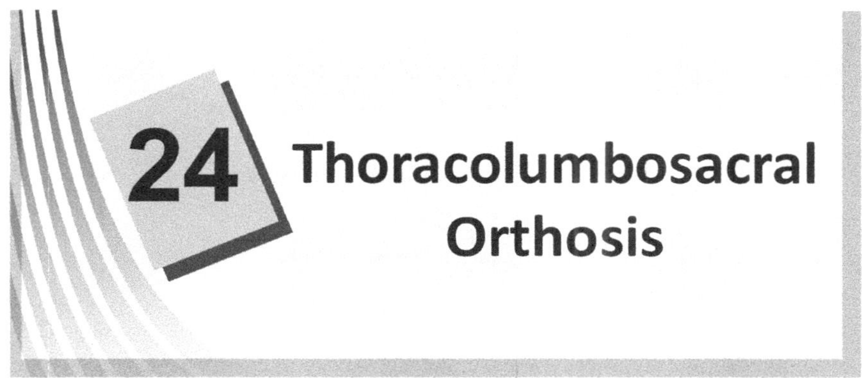

# 24 Thoracolumbosacral Orthosis

Support and immobilisation of thoracic and lumbar spines is achieved with the aid of a variety of orthosis grouped as thoracolumbar spinal orthosis.

Application of orthosis has three purposes:

1. Effectiveness of abdominal musculature in raising intra-abdominal pressure is enhanced by abdominal supports or corsets.
2. Range of movement is reduced.
3. Skeletal alignment is modified as per need of the pathology.

**Advantages**

1. Pain decreases by restriction of movement
2. Increased abdominal pressure reduces strain in lumbar disk
3. Modifications of skeletal alignment.

**Disadvantage**

1. Weakness due to reduced functional demand
2. Muscular atrophy following disuse
3. Contracture following immobilisation and atrophy
4. Psychological dependence.

**Principle**

Application of force to reduce movement is on the basis of three point pressure system. One pressure and two counter pressure. Arrows are pressure and counter pressure. Straight line shows change in alignment.

## LUMBOSACRAL ORTHOSIS

1. Lumbosacral belt
2. Lumbosacral corset
3. Lumbosacral anteroposterior control brace (Knight's brace)
4. Lumbosacral anteroposterolateral control brace (Chair back brace)
5. Lumbosacral posterolateral control brace (William's back brace).

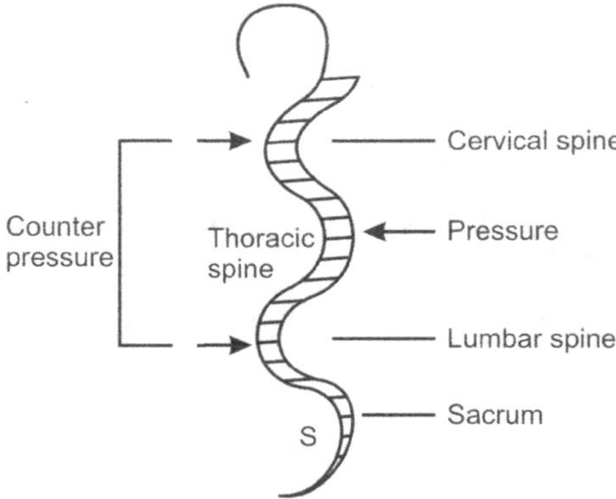


**Fig. 24.1:** 3-point pressure system used in correction of thoracic spine deformities. The block arrows represent the direction of force applied or excited by the orthosis. For correction of a deformity, pressure is applied over the deformity and correction is maintained by counter pressure from the opposite side.

## Chair Back Brace (LS APL Control Brace)

It controls flexion, extension and lateral bending. It consists anterior corset or straps with two posterior paraspinal uprights to limit flexion and extension and two uprights in mid axillary line to limit lateral bending.

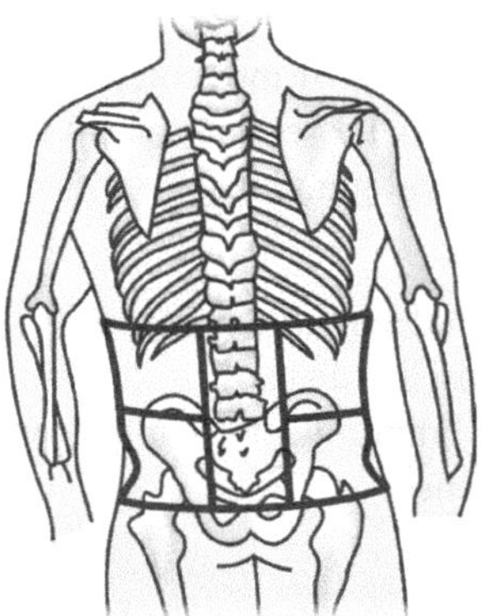

**Fig. 24.2:** Chair Back Lumbosacral Orthosis: Made of 2 posterior paraspinal uprights and anterior corset to limit flexion, extension. It also has 2 lateral uprights at midaxillary line to limit lateral bending.

It provides three-point pressure system (Figs 24.1 and 24.2):

1. Posteriorly directed pressure from anterior corset or straps that increases the abdominal pressure.
2. Anteriorly directed pressure from:
   a. Thoracic support
   b. Pelvic part on back.

## Knight's Brace (LS AP Control Brace)

It restricts extension and flexion but allows lateral flexion. It consists of pelvic band and thoracic band closed by straps. Both are connected posteriorly by two paraspinal uprights and laterally by two lateral uprights. Anteriorly it has a corset or anterior abdominal support (Fig. 24.3 A).

The three point pressures to prevent flexion are:

1. Anteriorly directed force from uprights
2. Posteriorly directed force from pelvic strap
3. Posteriorly directed force from thoracic strap.

The three point pressure to prevent extension are:

1. Posteriorly directed force from abdominal support
2. Anteriorly directed force from pelvic band
3. Anteriorly directed force from thoracic band.

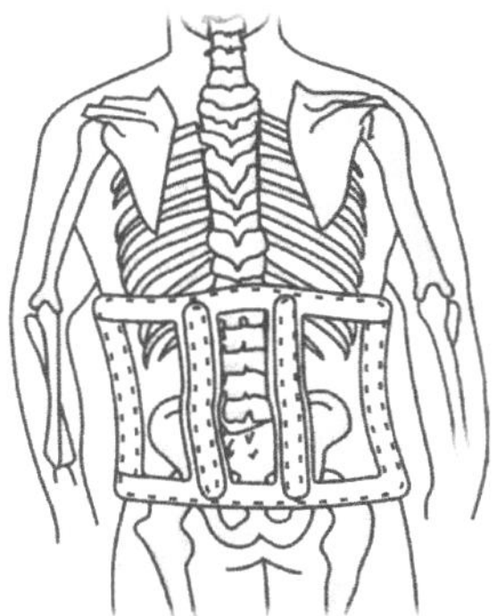

**Fig. 24.3A:** Knight's Brace: Made of pelvic band and thoracic band closed by straps. It has two paraspinal and two lateral uprights. Anteriorly it has a corset.

### *Indications*

1. Lumbar spondylosis
2. Lumbosacral strain
3. Osteoporosis
4. Acute disk lesions.

## William's Brace (LS PL Control Brace)

It restricts extension and flexion but allows lateral flexion. It has a lateral oblique upright that restricts lateral bending. It restricts extension by posteriorly directed force from abdominal corset and anteriorly directed force from pelvic and thoracic band (Fig. 24.3 B).

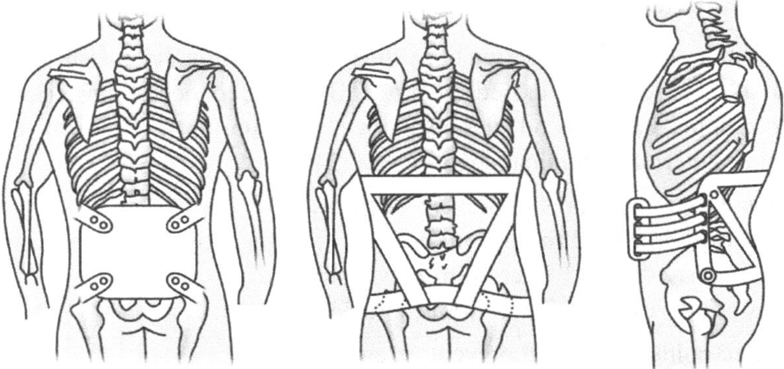

Fig. 24.3B: William's Brace: Has a pelvic band and thoracic band connected together by oblique lateral uprights.

## THORACOLUMBOSACRAL ORTHOSIS (TLSO) (FIGS 24.4 TO 24.6)

1. Taylor's orthosis
2. Chair back brace with sternal pad attachments
3. Molded plastic jackets
4. Jewett hyperextension orthosis

### Taylor's Brace (Fig. 24.5)

It consists of:

1. Two thoracic lumbar posterior uprights
2. Pelvic band

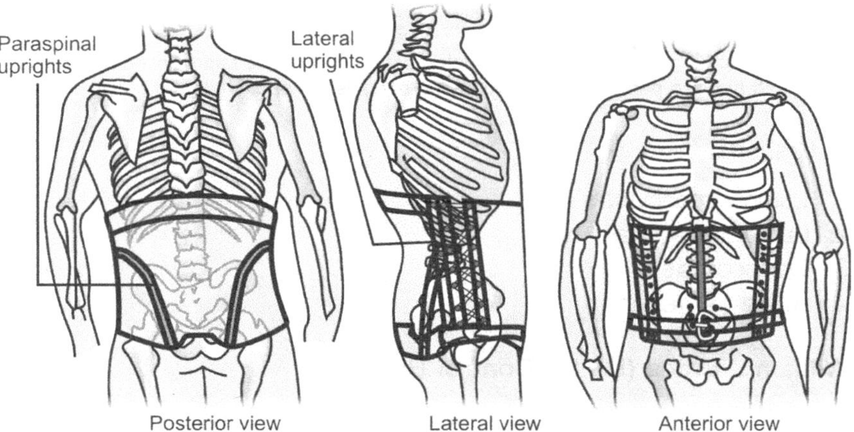


Fig. 24.4: Lumbosacral P and L Control Brace: Fabricated with posterior paraspinal metal uprights and lateral metal uprights to limit extension and lateral flexion. Anterior abdominal corset is made of canvas or leather.

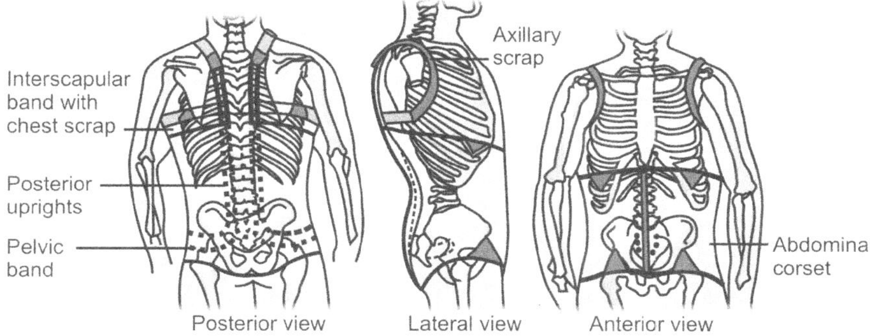


**Fig. 24.5:** Taylor's Brace: A thoracolumbo sacral orthosis which has paraspinal uprights from cervicothoracic junction till sacrum, pelvic band, interscapular band with chest strap, axillary strap, abdominal corset.

3. Interscapular band with chest strap
4. Axillary strap
5. Abdominal corset or straps.

The two uprights are attached inferiorly to pelvic band. The interscapular band stabilizes the upright and serves as attachment for axillary strap. Abdominal corsets or supports decreases the force applied to spine by converting abdominal cavity into a rigid chamber.

Three point pressure system to limit flexion:

a. Posteriorly directed force from pelvic strap
b. Posteriorly directed force from chest straps and axillary straps
c. Anteriorly directed force from upright.

Three point pressure to limit hyperextension:

a. Posteriorly directed force from corset or abdominal support
b. Anteriorly directed from pelvic band
c. Anteriorly directed force from posterior upright.

## Chair Back Brace with Sternal Attachment

Chair back brace is a modified TLSO with posteriorly directed forces by sternal plate instead of axillary and chest straps.

### *Advantages*

1. Increased comfort
2. Free arm.

### *Disadvantages*

1. Bulk in chest.
2. Decreases chest expansion.

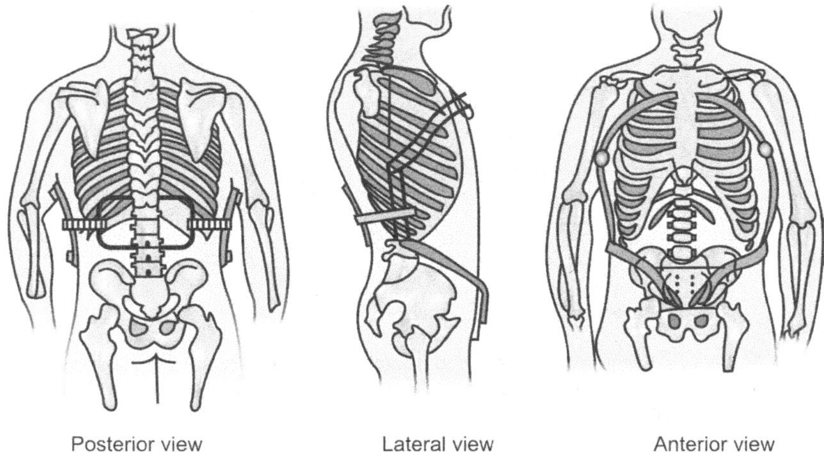


**Fig. 24.6:** Thoracolumbar anterior control brace

## Moulded Plaster Jacket

The jacket conforms to the contour of the body. It is a total contact orthosis with uniform pressure distribution and provides more support. It restricts spinal flexion, extension better than other braces.

## Jewett Hyperextension Orthosis

It is a thoracolumbar anterior control brace. It keeps spine in extension and prevents flexion.

Three point pressure that prevents flexion are:

1. Sternal support pad anteriorly
2. Suprapubic pad anteriorly
3. Thoracolumbar pad posteriorly used in compression fracture of thoracolumbar region.

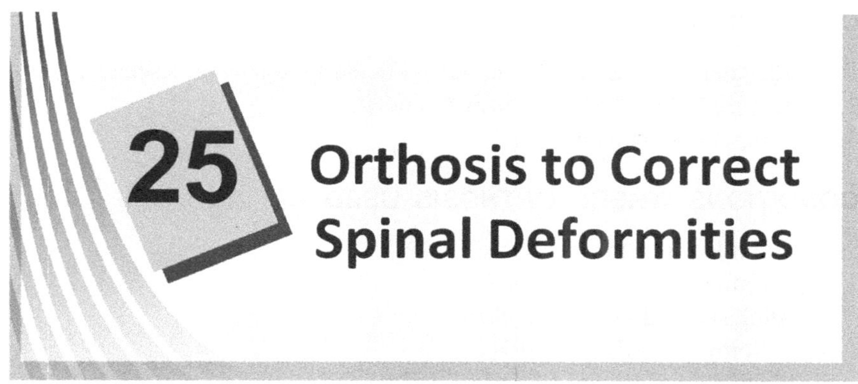

# 25 Orthosis to Correct Spinal Deformities

Scoliosis is a non physiological lateral curving of spine from mid line. To start with scoliosis is classified as:

a. Functional or mobile scoliosis that is reversible and disappears on recumbent posture.
b. Structural or fixed scoliosis: Is a fixed curve that does not correct itself on forward bending.

## INDICATIONS FOR NON-OPERATIVE TREATMENT

1. Young child with potential for growth.
2. In children up to 60° curve and adults up to 45° can be managed with brace.
3. Mild to moderate hump (less than 5 cm hump)
4. *Pattern of curve:*
   a. *Multiple small curve:*
      - Progress very little
      - Watch for 6 months
      - If increases use brace
   b. *Right thoracic:*
      - Good prognosis
   c. *Double major (thoracic and lumbar):*
      - Usually well compensated up to 40°
      - Brace is used. More than 60° surgical correction.
   e. *Double thoracic:* Well compensated Milwaukee brace to control.
5. Psychological and emotional stability to ensure proper usage of brace
6. Enthusiastic and supportive parents for proper treatment and continued follow up

## CONTRAINDICATIONS

1. Large lateral curves more than 60° particularly in late adolescence.
2. After epiphyses closed and growth ended.
3. Uncooperative patient.

## CONDITIONS WHERE ORTHOSIS USED

1. Infantile idiopathic scoliosis
2. Juvenile idiopathic scoliosis
3. Adolescent idiopathic scoliosis
4. Poliomyelitis with scoliosis
5. Meningomyelocele
6. Cerebral palsy
7. Traumatic spinal deformities
8. Spinal muscular atrophy
9. Congenital spinal deformity
10. Scheurmann's disease.

Orthosis not proved useful in muscular dystrophy, Fredrick's ataxia, congenital lordosis or congenital kyphosis.

## FACTORS FOR ORTHOSIS PRESCRIPTION

1. Degree, pattern and location of deformity
2. Progression of deformity
3. Age
4. Etiological factors
5. Motivation
6. Socioeconomic factors.

## FUNCTIONS OF CORRECTIVE ORTHOSIS

A. Prevents progression of curves
B. Improves structural alignment
    i. Reduces angulation and rotation
    ii. Improves trunk stability.
C. Reduces pain
D. Improves systemic function
E. Improves cosmesis.

## TYPES OF BRACES USED

1. Milwaukee brace
2. Thoracolumbosacral orthosis
3. Lumbosacral orthosis.

## Milwaukee Brace

Milwauhee brace is the first brace which had positive results in spinal deformity. It was designed in 1940 in Milwaukee by Blount and Schmidt. It was initially used to maintain corrected post surgical cases and later for non-operative treatment. It consist of four basic components (Fig. 25.1).

1. Pelvic mould or girdle
2. Head support unit
3. One anterior and two posterior uprights extending from pelvic girdle to head support.
4. Corrective pads.

### *Pelvic Girdle*

It is a leather or plastic pelvic mould and it extends anteriorly from tenth rib to a level above public symphysis and below Anterior Superior Iliac Spine (ASIS). Posteriorly from 10th rib to as low as possible with sitting clearance. This is foundation of entire brace and it provides reaction points for:

a. Vertical distraction forces
b. Corrective pads.

### *Head Support Unit*

It consists of:

a. Neck ring
b. A kidney shaped chin plate and
c. Butterfly shaped occipital plate. The uprights are attached with neck ring.

### *Uprights*

a. *Anterior:* It extends from a horizontal line through Anterior Superior Iliac Spine to chin.
b. Posterior para vertebral with 3 to 5 inches between. Extends between pelvic mould to neck ring.

### *Corrective Pads*

1. *Thoracic pad:* Is located on convex side of thoracic curve and it covers at least four ribs. It is connected by straps to anterior and posterior upright. It applies:
   a. Medial, superior and anterior directed force to vertebral column though ribs.
   b. Limits patient slump when fatigued
   c. Kinesthetic remainder to voluntarily move away from pad thus reducing the curve.
   d. It also serves as counter force to opposing pads like axillary pad.

2. *Axillary pad:* It covers pectoral, axillary and scapular areas. It provides
   a. Medially and superiorly directed force onside opposite to thoracic pad.
   b. It can retract, protract or elevate the shoulder girdle.
   c. Improves symmetry of shoulder girdle.
3. *Shoulder ring:* It covers pectoral, axillary, scapular and clavicular areas. It provides medial and inferiorly directed force. It helps to retract, protract or depress the shoulder girdle and thus improves symmetry of shoulder girdle.
4. *Lumbar plate:* Is used in lumbar curves and it provides anterior and medially directed force to lumbar spine. Assist in lumbar curves correction and deviation.
5. *Kyphosis pad:* Used to current kyphosis and is located over the apex of kyphosis, and attached to both posterior uprights. It provides anteriorly directed force at the apex of kyphosis curve. With sternal pad it helps in voluntary extension of upper thoracic and cervical spine.
6. *Sternal pad:* Located anterior to sternal notch. It encourages, voluntary extension of upper thoracic and cervical spine. It also relieves pressure at chin plate.

*Forces used to achieve correction:*

1. *Passive forces:*
   a. Longitudinal distraction force:
      - Vertical up ward traction from pelvis to skull.
   b. Anti-angulation and derotation force
      - Lateral bend against the curve.
      - Localized pressure at apex of curve

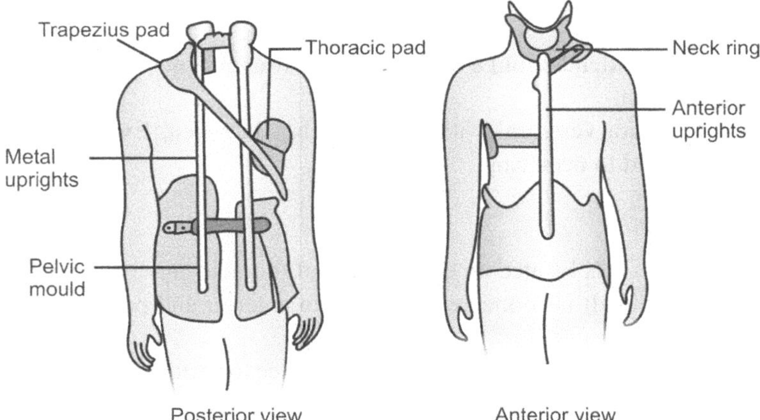


**Fig. 25.1:** Milwaukee Brace: A rigid corrective spinal orthosis which has a pelvic mould and head support unit. One anterior and two posterior uprights extend from pelvic girdle to head support. Corrective pads are applied appropriately using three-point pressure principle, i.e. one pressure and two counter pressure.

2. *Active forces:*
   a. Muscular exertion to move away from pressure of appliance
   b. Exercise program with or without appliance to maintain muscle tone.

## Complications

1. Deep sores from pressure on skin over bony prominence.
2. *Bite deformities:* Due to pressure of chin pad on mandible. It causes growth disturbances of jaw or teeth.
3. Exaggerated emotional disturbance and rejection of brace.

*Exercises to be done in Milwaukee brace*

1. Pelvic tilt supine with knee flexed
   a. Keep shoulders flat on floor and chest elevated and breathe regularly.
   b. Tighten buttock muscles
   c. Force lumbar spine towards floor by tightening and pushing backward the abdominal muscles.
2. Pelvic tilt supine with knee straight repeat a,b,c,
3. Pelvic tilt standing
   a. Relax knees, tilt the pelvis
   b. Stand tall elevate the chest and breathe regularly.
   c. Walk, holdup the tilt. Make this posture a habit.
4. Spine extension is prone position
   a. With knees held down tilt the pelvis
   b. Raise the shoulder about 3 inches against resistance between shoulder blades.
5. Push up with pelvis tilted.
6. Correction of thoracic lordosis and rib hump
   a. Tilt the pelvis in standing position
   b. Inhale deeply, and press the chest wall backward.
7. Active correction of major curve:
   a. Tilt the pelvis
   b. Keep the pelvis tilted and shift the torso to the right or left.

All the exercises to be performed and held for a count of five. Each exercise should be done ten times.

*Exercises out of Milwaukee brace:*

Each to be done for 5 counts and done for ten times:

1. Pelvic tilt supine with knee flexed:
   a. Keep shoulder flat on floor, chest elevated but breathe regularly
   b. Tighten buttock muscles
   c. Force the small back to floor by tightening, pushing backward the abdominal muscles.
2. Pelvic tilt with knee straight repeat a,b,c,

3. Sit up with pelvic tilt
   a. When knees flexed tilt the pelvis and hold the tilt.
   b. With elbows straight roll up to touch the knees with fingers.
   c. Roll back down slowly.
   d. Release the tilt.
4. Pelvis tilt in standing position
   a. With black against wall and heels 3 inches from wall, stand tall, elevate the chest but breathe regularly.
   b. Relax knee tilt the pelvis
   c. Walk away holding the tilt. Makes this as a habit.
5. Deep breathing exercises.
   a. Divide chest into three parts upper, middle and lower.
   b. Inhale deeply and exhale completely in each part.
6. Spine extension in prone position
   a. With knees held down tilt the pelvis
   b. Raise the shoulders about 3 inches firm against resistance between the shoulder blades.
7. Push up with the pelvis tilted.

## Thoracolumbosacral Orthosis

It extends from the level of axilla to the pelvis (Figs 25.2A and B).

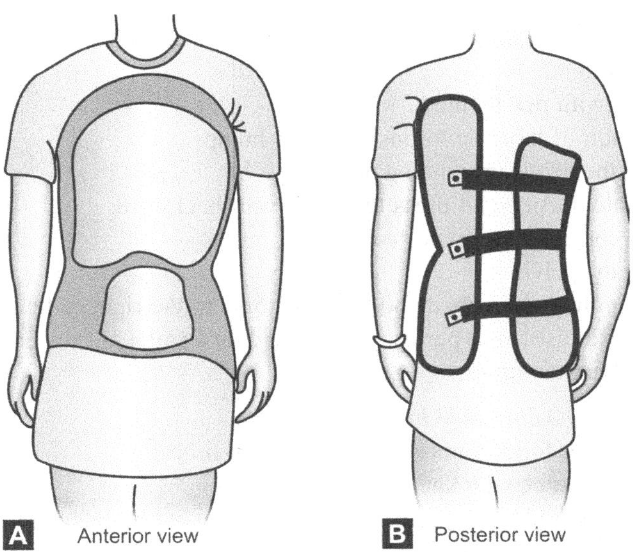


**Figs 25.2A and B:** Corrective thoracolumbo sacral orthosis
A. Anterior view shows the large anterior window to ease breathing movement of chest.
B. Posterior view shows custom made corrective pads and straps to correct spinal deformity.

*Indications*

a. Scoliosis with apex at T9 or lower
b. Kyphosis with apex at thoracolumbar junction.
Number of varieties of TLSO are available and they are named based on center at which it is made e.g. Lyon, Gillette, Boston.

## Lumbosacral Orthosis

Used only for lumbar scoliosis and it has a strong lumbar pad against apex of the curve. It is useful in idiopathic scoliosis.

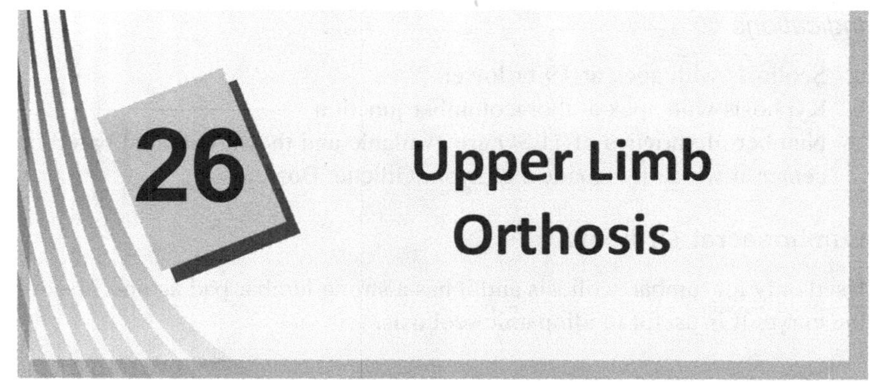


## PRINCIPLES IN APPLYING AN UPPER LIMB ORTHOSIS

1. Protection of an impaired joint or part by:
   a. Restricting the impaired joint thus maintaining the alignment and preventing deformity
   b. Stabilize the unstable bony components and promote healing of soft tissue and bones.
2. Correcting joint contractures, subluxation of joints or tendons thus reducing deformities
3. Assists in improving function by compensating for the deformity, muscle weakness and increased muscle tone.

## NAMING THE ORTHOSIS

1. By international standard organization of international society for prosthetics and orthotics, naming is done on the basis of the joints it encompasses and adding "o" at the end. It does not specify the function of orthosis.
2. ASHT SCS (American Society of Hand Therapists Splint Classification System) identifies orthosis in mobilization or immobilization or restriction. It also gives the direction of force applied. It also indicates the primary and secondary joint. Primarily is the one mainly affected by the orthosis. Secondary joints provides counter force, position or stabilization.

## CLASSIFICATION

1. Static
   a. Serial static
   b. Static motion blocking
   c. Static progressive

2. Dynamic
   a. Motion blocking
   b. Traction
   c. Tenodesis
3. Continuous Passive Motion Orthoses
4. Adaptive orthoses.

## • Static Orthoses: Serial Static Splint

A static splint but the angle of positioning is changed periodically. For example, in flexion contracture of wrist, with serial reposition splints, the range of movement can be improved.

### Static Motion Blocking Splint

Permits motion in one direction and blocks other movement. For example, swan neck splint blocks hyperextension and allows flexion at PIP joint.

### Static Progressive Splint

Used to regain range of motion. The joint is placed in a position of stretch and once motion is increased the tension is increased progressively.

## • Dynamic Orthoses: Dynamic Motion Blocking

Utilizes passive elastic pull in one direction and active movement in the other direction. This allows to maintain the functioning of the unaffected group of muscles. For example, dynamic cock up splint, active flexion and passive extension is allowed.

### Dynamic Traction Splints

It offers traction to a joint and allows controlled movement only.

### Tenodesis Splint

Utilizes active extension of wrist in C6 tetraplegic patient to produce controlled passive flexion of fingers against a static thumb post using the principle of parallelogram.

## • Continuous Passive Motion Orthosis

Electrically operated devices that moves the joints in the desired preprogrammed range of movement.

## STATIC ARM ORTHOSIS

### Shoulder and Arm Orthosis

1. *Slings–figure of 8 orthosis:* It is used to support shoulder, elbow and forearm. This helps in preventing subluxation of shoulder in hemiplegia, tetraplegia.
2. *Air-plane splint:* It keeps the arm in 90° abduction and allows no movement in the glenohumeral joint. It is made of plastic or metal and it is held to the chest wall by straps or elastic bandage. Indicated in Erb's palsy and burns in the axilla.

### Elbow Orthosis

1. *Static positioning elbow orthosis:* To hold a damaged or unstable joint in alignment.
2. *Static elbow wrist orthosis:* It immobilizes elbow, forearm and wrist in functional position. Commonly used in post burns rehabilitation.

### Wrist Orthosis

1. *Volar orthosis:*
   Cock up splint
   Volar Wrist Hand Orthoses
2. *Dorsal wrist orthosis:*
   Long opponens splint
   Dorsal WHO

### Hand and Finger Orthosis

1. Short opponens orthosis (Fig. 26.1)
2. Bennet type of metal hand orthosis
3. Rancho static orthosis with opponens bar, "C" bar and volar strap

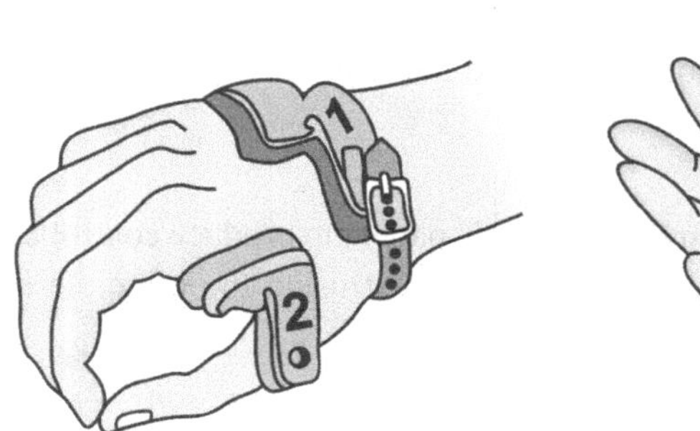


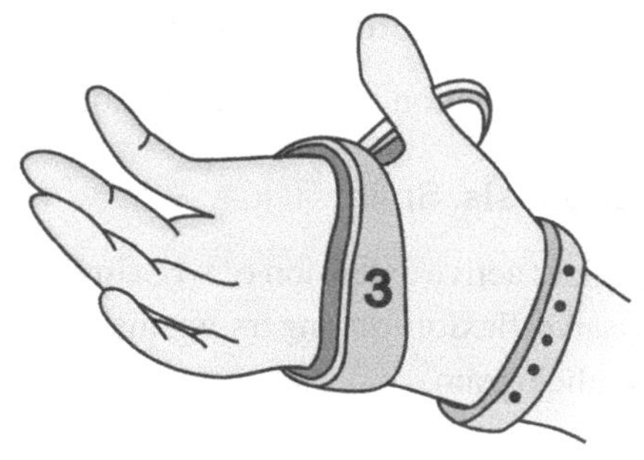


Short opponens hand splint

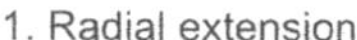

1. Radial extension
2. Thumb opposition
3. Palmar arch

**Fig. 26.1:** Short opponens splint maintains wrist in radical extension (corrects ulnar deviation), a opponens bar (thumb in abduction and internal rotation) and a palmar arch.

## Finger Orthosis

a. Static:
   1. Boutonniere orthosis (Fig. 26.2)
   2. Swan neck orthosis
   3. Mallet finger orthosis

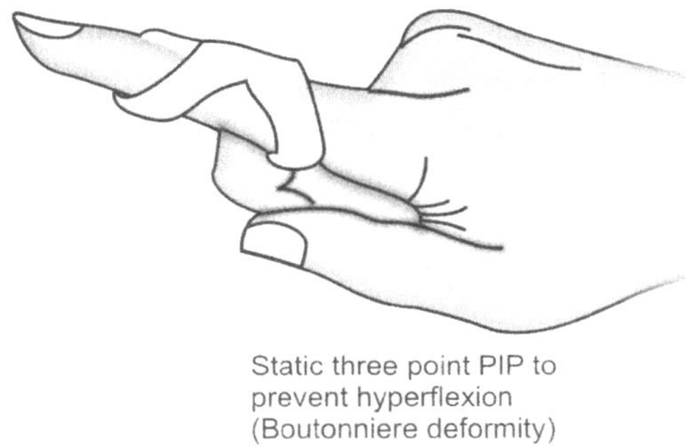


**Fig. 26.2:** Boutonniere splint: A static splint corrects hyperflexion at PIP joint by 3-point pressure principle.

## DYNAMIC ORTHOSIS

## Shoulder Orthosis

1. *Balanced forearm orthosis:* It is the most useful device to assist both elbow and shoulder function. It can be mounted on a wheelchair or on a table or occasionally on a belt at the level of iliac crest. It consists of a trough in which the proximal forearm rests. A pivot and linkage system under the trough is adjusted and preset so that the patient learn to produce movement at elbow and shoulder, with the movements of trunk and shoulder girdle.

## Elbow Orthosis

1. Functional dynamic elbow flexion orthosis.
2. Functional dynamic elbow extension orthosis.

## Wrist Orthosis

1. *Dynamic wrist orthosis with dorsiflexion assist:* It is a modified long opponens splint designed to assist wrist extension and allowing normal flexion of wrist.

## Dynamic Hand Orthosis

- To substitute for absent or weak extension.
- Wrist extension finger flexion reciprocal orthosis (Flexor Hinge Splint).

## Hand and Finger Orthosis

1. Metacarpophalangeal flexion orthosis to prevent the metacarpophalangeal extension.
2. Metacarpophalangeal extension orthosis for finger drop.
3. PIP extension stop
4. PIP flexion stop
5. *Thumb IP extension assist:* Indicated in finger and thumb drop in radial nerve or posterior interosseus nerve injury.
6. *First dorsal interosseus assist:* Keeps the index finger abducted and in opposition.

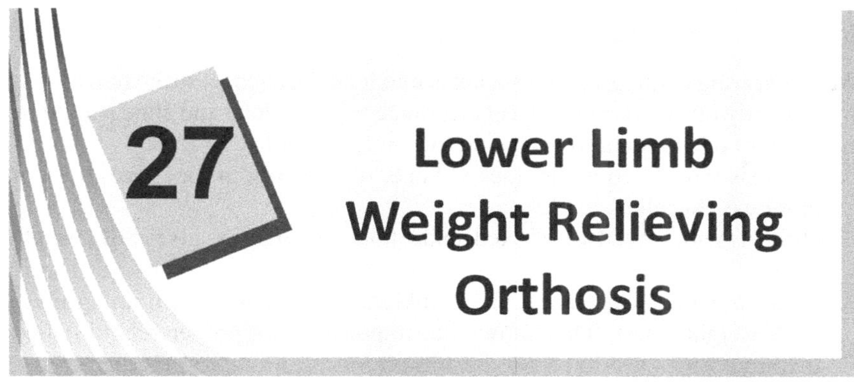

# 27 Lower Limb Weight Relieving Orthosis

## WEIGHT RELIEVING ORTHOSIS

The weight of the limb is taken by the orthosis and relieves the weight bearing stress on the skeletal structures. Commonly used are:

1. Ischial weight relieving orthosis
2. PTB weight relieving orthosis.

### Ischial Weight Relieving Orthosis

It is designed to transmit force from ischium to orthosis and through orthosis to ground. It consists of:

a. *Ischial weight bearing area:* Ischial seat bears weight like in quadrilateral socket of above knee prosthesis.
b. Stainless steel bar connected to external knee joint and connected to bottom by a stirrup. The stirrup is riveted to sole plate extending to metatarsal head with boot or rocker-bottom boot (Fig. 27.1).

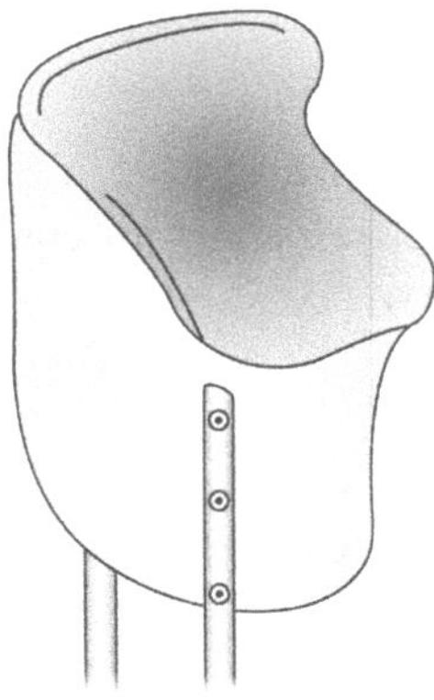

**Fig. 27.1:** Quadrilateral hollow socket with ischial seat

### *Biomechanical Principle*

Weight bearing in quadrilateral socket is maximal during heel strike but it drops significantly during push off. Heel clearance between heel and shoe should be a minimum of 3/8 inch, to give effective weight relief.

1. Orthosis with fixed ankle, locked knee, rocker bottom foot gives 90% or more weight relief.
2. Orthosis with locked knee, fixed ankle, boot with training gives 86% weight relief.
3. Orthosis with locked knee, fixed ankle, and boot without training gives 60% weight relief. This shows the importance of proper rehabilitation therapy.

### *Indications*

1. Perthe's disease
2. Slipped femoral epiphysis
3. TB hip
4. Fractures of femur with non-union
5. Severe osteoarthritis hip.

## Patellar Tendon Bearing Weight Relieving Orthosis

Transmits the force from knee through patellar tendon through the uprights and shoe to the ground. For easy donning and doffing PTB cuff is bivalved and closed by rigid buckles or straps. The cuff should be in 10° flexion for effective weight bearing. Fixed ankle should be in 7 to 10° dorsiflexion. The best results are achieved with:

a. Fixed ankle
b. One inch heel clearance
c. Rocker bottom shoe.

### *Indications for PTB Weight Relieving Orthosis*

*Short-term:*

1. Healing of fracture calcaneum
2. Postoperative fusion about ankle
3. Painful condition of heel refractory to conservative management and contraindicated to surgery.

*Long-term:*

1. Delayed non-union fractures of tibia
2. Avascular necrosis of body of talus
3. Severe degenerative arthritis of ankle and subtalar joints
4. Osteomyelitis of calcaneum
5. Diabetic ulceration foot
6. Sciatic nerve injury with insensitive sole of foot
7. Chronic and painful conditions that are not amenable to surgery.

# 28 Lower Limb Orthosis

The major classification in lower limb orthoses are:

1. Foot orthoses—FO
2. Ankle foot orthoses—AFO
3. Knee ankle foot orthoses—KAFO
4. Hip knee ankle foot orthoses—HKAFO
5. HKAFO with spinal support.

## PRINCIPLES IN LOWER LIMB ORTHOSES

1. Use only as indicated and as long necessary
2. Allow joint movement where ever possible
3. Orthosis should be functional in all phases of gait
4. Orthotic ankle should be centered over tip of medial malleolus
5. Orthotic knee joint should be centered over prominence of medial femoral condyle
6. Orthotic hip joint should be in a position that allows patient to sit upright Usually 1/4 inch anterior and 1/4 inch superior to greater trochanter
7. It should be comfortable
8. Cosmetic
9. Cheap and easy to maintain.

## ANKLE FOOT ORTHOSIS

Mostly commonly prescribed orthosis in lower limb. It can provide.

1. Mediolateral stability in ankle and preventing twisting of ankle during stance
2. Provides toe pick up during swing to prevent dragging of toe
3. Push off simulation during late stance
4. Can be used to correct valgus/varus deformities.

AFO may be metal or plastic AFO.

## Metal AFO

It consists of:

a. Calf band
b. Metal uprights
c. Ankle joint
d. Stirrup
e. Sole plate
f. Boot.

### *Calf Band*

Calf band is given proximally at one inch below fibular neck, 1½ to 3 inch in breadth closed anteriorly by straps.

### *Metal Uprights*

Two metal uprights are used in most orthoses. Single posterior upright can also be used, but it will not provide adequate ankle stability.

### *Ankle Joints*

1. Fixed ankle—no movement. Used with weight relieving orthoses
2. Free ankle—plantar flexion, dorsiflexion, inversion and eversion is allowed. Commonly used with KAFO or HKAFO when the power in foot and ankle is normal
3. *Limited ankle:* 10° dorsiflexion 10° plantar flexion allowed. Used in flail foot
4. *Ankle with foot drop stop:* Used in weakness of dorsiflexors with over action of plantar flexors.
   a. Provides toe pick up and helps toe clearance. Thus preventing toe drag and tumbling.
   b. Creating a bending moment at knee.

   The Flexion moment at knee can be prevented by:
   - Good knee extensors which can compensate the flexion moment
   - FDS with 5° plantar flexion reduces bending moment
   - Use of a cushion heel like SACH foot.
5. *Ankle with dorsiflexion stop:* With weak plantar flexors with overacting dorsiflexors with calcaneo deformity it is indicated.
   a. Orthosis helps to keep foot flat
   b. With a sole plate extending beyond metatarsal head, as the heel raises the shoe pivots over sole plate simulating a push off.

c. The pivoting of shoe over sole plate causes extension moments providing knee stability.

### *Stirrup*

Stirrup is a "U" shaped metal attached to the shoe. It side ends are bent to form a part of ankle joints medial and lateral.

### *Sole Plate*

Extension of stirrup into sole.

## Metal AFO for Valgus Deformity

'T' straps along the side of shoe distal to subtalar joint. Medial or inside 'T' strap to control valgus deformity (Fig. 28.1 A).

## AFO with Varus

Lateral or outside 'T' strap to control varus deformity.

## Plastic AFO

The foot extends beyond metatarsal head. It can be a custom made matching each patient. The AFO can be made more stable by (Fig. 28.1 B):

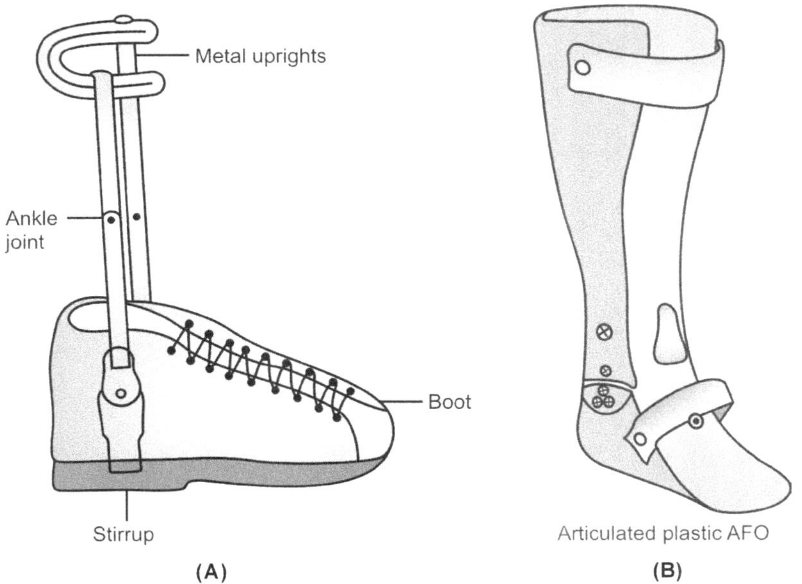


**Figs 28.1A and B:** (A) Metal AFO : Most commonly used orthosis. Made of calf band, medical and lateral uprights, ankle joint, stirrup with boot. (B) Articulated Plastic AFO : Made of hard plastic and custom made to each patient. Has an ankle joint-single axis which allows limited plantar flexion and dorsiflexion.

a. The trim line extends more anteriorly
b. Thicker layer of plastic
c. Medial and lateral carbon inserts
d. Corrugations in posterior leaf.

AFO can be also be provided with hinge joints which can allow full or partial motions. Energy consumption with metal or plastic AFO is same but the weight is less.

## KNEE ANKLE FOOT ORTHOSIS (KAFO)

Knee Ankle Foot Orthosis: Made up of medical and lateral uprights, upper and lower thigh bands, knee joint with drop lock, calf band, ankle joint, stirrup with boot. The type of knee joint and ankle joint varies according to the indication of orthosis (Fig. 28.2).

It provides:

1. Knee stability in cases where AFO is not adequate. *Knee stability:* is achieved by three point principle. Stabilizing force is applied is the anterior knee support. The thigh band and calf band or at shoe level are the counters acting forces.
2. Mediolateral stability at ankle.
3. Simulated push off if filted with dorsiflexion stop with sole plate extending to metatarsal head.
4. With foot drop stop it provides toe clearance.

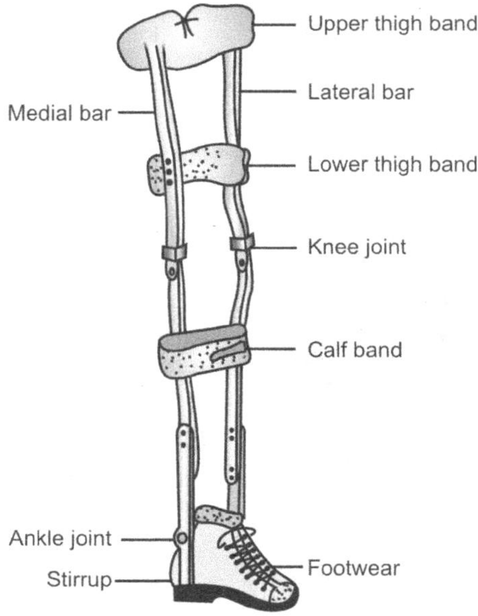


**Fig. 28.2:** Knee ankle foot orthosis

## Parts of KAFO

1. Thigh uprights medial and lateral
2. Proximal and or lower thigh band
3. Knee joint
4. Anterior knee support
5. Leg uprights
6. Ankle joint
7. Stirrup
8. Sole plate
9. 'T' straps
10. Shoes.

### *Thigh Band*

1. Upper thigh band 1½ inch below ischium, closed anteriorly by strap
2. Lower thigh band with soft front closure is also used.

### *Knee Joints*

Various types of knee joints used in orthosis are as follows (Fig. 28.3):

1. Straight set knee commonly used. It allows free flexion but restricts hyper-extension. Used with a drop lock. It keeps the knee extended in all phases of gait.
2. *Polycentric knee:* In addition it allows rotation of tibia over femur, mostly used in sport knee orthoses.
3. *Offset knee:* Posterior offset knee is indicated with weak quadriceps and good hip extensor. It keeps the ground reaction force in front of knee thus reducing knee flexion moment and creating an extension moment and stabilizes knee.

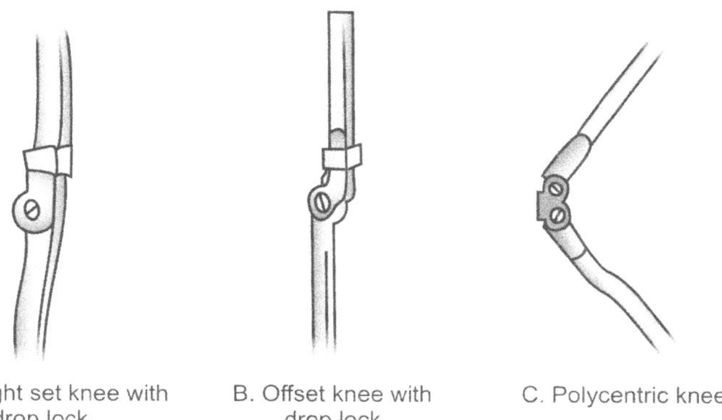

A. Straight set knee with drop lock B. Offset knee with drop lock C. Polycentric knee

**Fig. 28.3:** Types of joints in orthosis

*Knee Locks*

1. Drop lock (commonly used)
2. Bail lock.

*Anterior Knee Supports (Fig. 28.4)*

1. Knee cap
2. Patellar tendon strap
3. Suprapatellar strap
4. Suprapatellar and patellar tendon strap

Out of four combinations supra patellar strap and PTB strap is best suitable as it is over pressure resistant area. The ankle joints and shoe are the same like AFO.

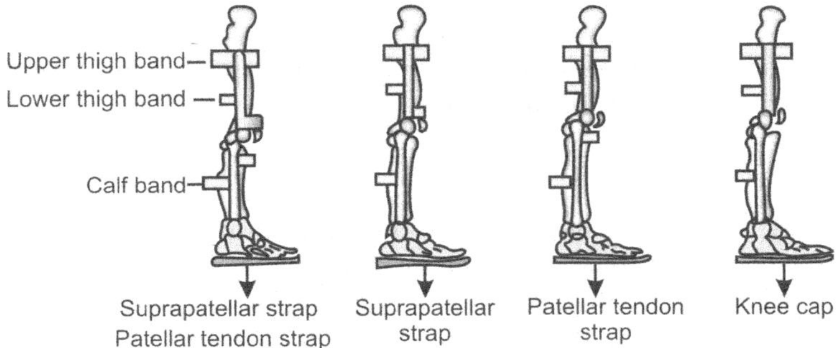


**Fig. 28.4:** Types of anterior knee supports

## HIP KNEE ANKLE FOOT ORTHOSIS (HKAFO)

It is given when the hip muscles are weak; especially hip abductors and with hip instability. It has external hip joint and in addition pelvic band to stabilize the hip.

### HKAFO with Spinal Support

It can be given for patients with spinal extensor weakness. Patient needs assistive device to ambulate.

### Functional Cast Bracing

In the treatment of lower extremity fractures, patellar tendon bearing and ischial weight bearing design have been used.

*Advantages*

1. Immobilization period is reduced
2. Decreased incidence of delayed or non union.

It's success is due to:
a. Maintaining bone alignment
b. Limit weight bearing through fracture site to a tolerable level.
c. Early ambulation.

## Seattle Ort\hosis

The first plastic orthoses made and described. It is rigid and it encases ankle. It is equal to AFO with anterior and posterior pin stop with sole plate extending to metatarsal head area. It also provides good mediolateral stability.

## Berkeley Dual Ankle Orthosis

It is based on the principle that the axis of inversion and eversion of subtalar joint is at 42° from horizontal plane and 23° from midline of foot. Orthosis is designed with axis located posteriorly to the heel of the shoe to allow inversion and eversion.

## Craig Scott Orthosis

It is an orthosis given to paraplegic with neurological level L1 or above. It is a modified KAFO of:
a. Lighter weight
b. East donning and doffing.

It consists of:
a. Ankle joint with anterior and posterior stop
b. Sole plate extending to metatarsal heads and with cross bar
c. Offset knee joint with bail lock
d. Rigid anterior tibial band positioned below tibial tubercle
e. Rigid posterior thigh band with soft closure anteriorly.

The three point system to keep knee in extension is:
1. Proximal thigh band posteriorly
2. Calcaneum posteriorly
3. Tibial band anteriorly.

## Swivel Orthosis or Para Podium

Is an orthosis given to children between 2½ to 5 years of age who are unlikely to become functional walkers due to severe impairment. The child moves by pivoting the hips to swivel to one side of oval based stand forward. The child repeats the same with other leg. It has hip and knee joints that is kept locked during ambulation but unlocked for sitting.

## Reciprocating Gait Orthosis

Formerly known as hip guidance orthosis. It is a bilateral HKAFO (Fig. 28.5).

### *Principle*

Ipsilateral hip flexion leads to contralateral hip extension and *vice versa*. It consists of a hip joint that transfer forces from one hip to other by Bowden cables. It is indicated in:

1. Children with active hip flexion and no hip extension.
2. Paraplegic L1 level with active hip flexion and no extension.

It lost its fame due to:

1. High energy requirement
2. Slow speed

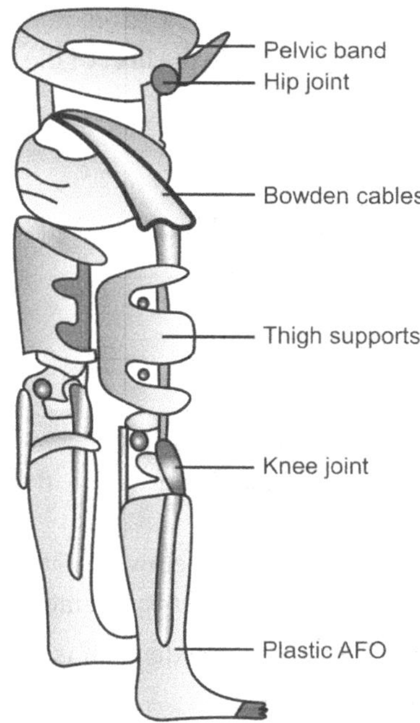


**Fig. 28.5:** Reciprocating Gait Orthosis: Modified Hip Knee Ankle Foot Orthosis with a Bowden cable system to transfer force from one hip to other hip to produce reciprocating pattern of walking.

## Knee Cage

It is used for genu recurvatum. Two types of knee cage is prescribed commonly. They differ based on principle of action.

a. Swedish knee cage
b. Madras knee cage

*a. Swedish Knee Cage*

It is used to control mild to moderate recurvatum due to ligamentous or capsular laxity. Maybe of:

1. Non-articulated variety– Does not allow knee flexion or extension.
2. Articulated variety– Allows full knee flexion and prevents hyperextension it is based on three points principle (Fig. 28.6).

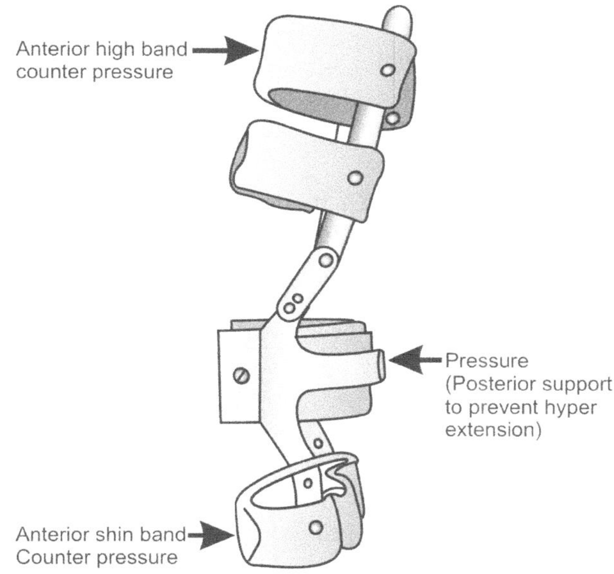


**Fig. 28.6:** Swedish knee cage (Articulated type)

*b. Madras Knee Cage*

It is also prescribed for genu recurvatum. One superior pressure at supra-patellar bursa level and other below neck of fibula posteriorly and a mechanical knee joint helps in reducing genu recurvatum.

## Solid Plastic AFO

This resists plantar flexion which can produce knee flexion moment at knee thus preventing recurvatum. The flexion moment can be increased by AFO with dorsiflexion.

## Floor Reaction Orthosis

It is a modified AFO which not only provides ankle stability but helps in knee stability by providing knee extension moment.

### Principle

Foot is kept in pla ntar flexion as the heel is 1 cm above the ground. On initial contact (with forefoot instead of normal heel strike) a turning moment is created at the ankle which accenterates the knee extension moment at stance leading to stability at knee.

### Results

a. Stabilization of ankle
b. Stabilization of subtalar joint
c. Assists in knee stability.

### Types (Fig. 28.7)

1. *Single unit floor reaction AFO:* It consists of a single unit plastic AFO with foot in plantar flexion and proximal anterior stabilization with steel.

*Advantages:* Lighter, close fitting and easy to fabricate.

*Disadvantage:* Foot and leg has to be inserted through the opening so difficult to wear.

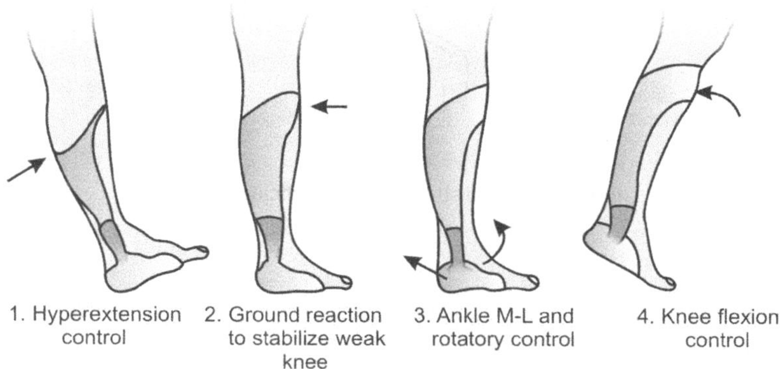


**Fig. 28.7:** Ground reaction AFO dynamic illustration

2. *Extendable floor reaction orthosis:* It is separated proximally into medial and lateral parts. It can also be extended lengthwise. So it is useful in growing children.

3. *Rear entry floor reaction AFO:* It is an articulated AFO. It extends proximally more and foot is covered circumferentially. It allows heel strike and plantar flexion and prevents dorsiflexion. This prevents knee flexion. It is easy to donn and doff.

*Indications for Floor Reaction Orthosis*

1. Poliomyelitis with weakness in foot and ankle with inadequate quadriceps for knee stability
2. Cerebral palsy with knee flexion in stance phase
3. Meningomyelocele
4. Paraparesis.

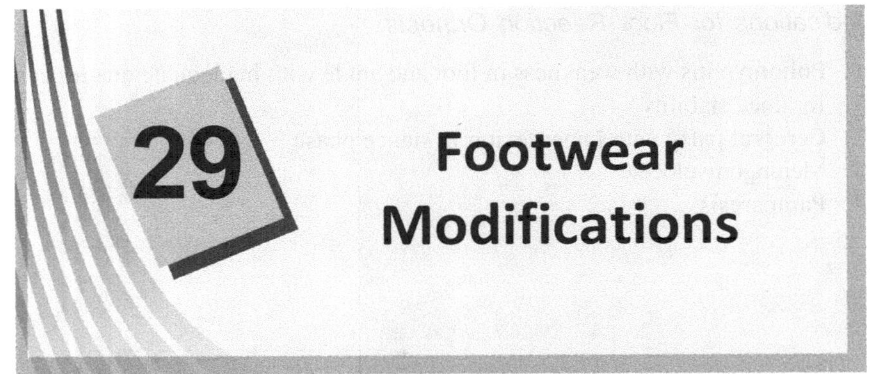

# 29 Footwear Modifications

The main purpose of wearing chappal, sandals, shoes and boots is to protect the feet. Presence of calluses indicates a friction from poorly fitting shoes. Corn indicates friction over bony points. Leather shoes are better because of the following characteristics:

1. Durable
2. Allow ventilation
3. Moulds to feet with time.

## PARTS OF SHOES (Fig. 29.1)

### Lower Part

1. Sole is made of leather or rubber
2. Shank is narrow part of sole between heel and ball
3. Ball is the widest part of sole in metatarsal region
4. Toe spring is the space between outer sole and floor. Helps to produce rocker effect during toe off
5. Heel helps to stuff the weight to forefoot.

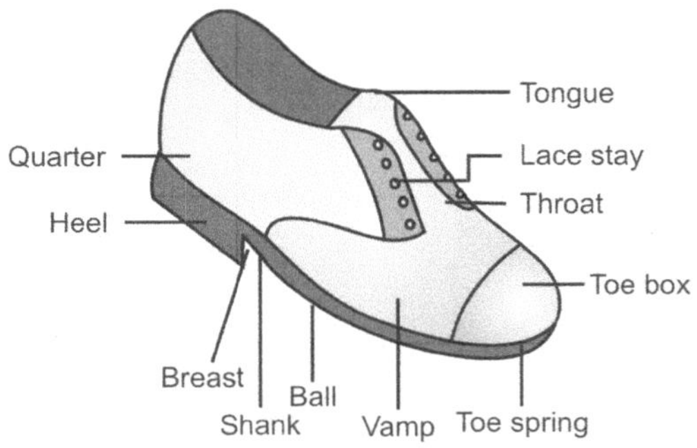


**Fig. 29.1:** Parts of normal shoe

### Upper Part

1. Quarter is the posterior portion of upper part and connected with heel counter
2. Heel counter provides posterior stability to shoe. With quarter, heel counter supports calcaneum
3. Vamp is anterior portion of upper part
4. Toe box is a extreme part of vamp that protects toes from trauma
5. Tongue is cover attached to vamp
6. Throat is the entrance of shoe.

## FOOT ORTHOSES

The effectiveness of orthosis depends on:

a. Proper diagnosis of condition.
b. Selection of appropriate orthotic materials
c. Proper molding.

Common condition where orthosis used are:

1. Pes planus
2. Pes cavus
3. Metatarsalgia
4. Heel pain
5. Toe pain
6. Limb length discrepancy
7. Insensitive foot
8. Osteoarthritis knee
9. Club foot
10. Boots for amputations.

### • Pes Planus (Flat Foot)

Pes planus is reduction in medial arch of foot with lowering of medial aspect of foot. The foot may be of planovalgus position. Pes planus consists of pronation and abduction of foot at subtalar joint. Pronation can be controlled by keeping subtalar joint in neutral position. Flat foot maybe (a) flexible and (b) rigid flat foot.

#### *Flexible Flat Foot*

In flexible flat foot, the collapse of medial arch occurs only on weight bearing. It results in pronated foot with longitudinal arch strain.

Footwear Modification:

1. *Thomas heel shoe* has heel extension on medial side up to a part of medial arch with long medial counter (Figs 29.2 A and B).

2. *Medial arch supports:* Height of arch has to be increased as necessary as the foot develops tolerance.
3. Custom molded foot orthosis with elevation of anteromedial calcaneum (exerts upward thrust against sustentaculum tali thus preventing in rolling). This orthosis is also called as UCBL (University of California Biomechanics Laboratory)
4. Thomas heel with medial heel wedge useful for children with flexible flat foot. Wedge is of 1/16 inch up to 2 years of age and 1/8 up to five years and 3/10 inch after five years.

### *Rigid Flat Foot*

In rigid flat foot, collapse occurs both on weight bearing and non-weight bearing. Should not be filled with arch supports or Thomas Heel. Here foot wear modification is done only for pain relief and not for correction of deformity.

## FOOTWEAR MODIFICATION

A molded polyurethane foam backed by microcellular rubber can provide good comfort to sole

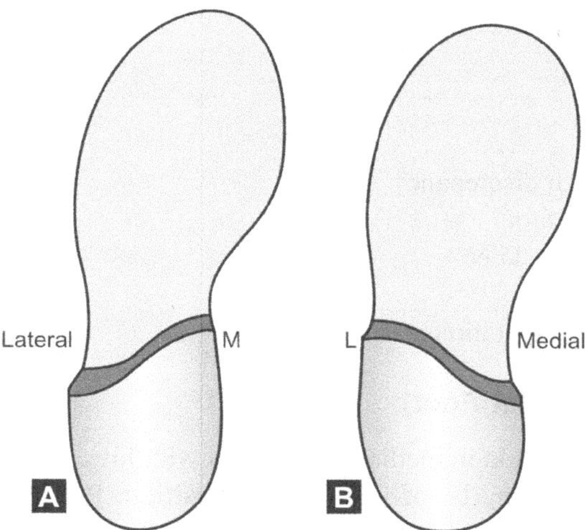


**Figs 29.2A and B:** A. Thomas heel : Has a heel extended anteriorly on the medial side. B. Reverse thomas heel : Has heel extended anteriorly on the lateral side.

## Pes Cavus

Pes cavus is a high arched foot which leads to excess pressure along heel and metatarsal head areas.

Footwear modification:

1. *In case of high arch without supination:* Longitudinal arch support to fill the space between shoe and arch and it is extended to metatarsal heads.

2. *If the foot is supinated and lateral aspect bears more weight:* Custom made foot orthosis with subtalar joint in neutral position has to be used.

• **Metatarsalgia:** Metatarsalgia is defined as painful metatarsal heads due to uneven distribution of weight.

Pain is relieved by distributing weight proximal to metatarsal head thus reducing the stress on metatarsal heads. This can be done with internal or external modification.

Footwear modification:

1. Metatarsal pad (Fig. 29.3) is fixed inside the shoe, posterior to 2nd, 3rd, 4th metatarsal head lateral to metatarsal head of big toe medial to metatarsal head of little toe.
2. Metatarsal bar (Fig. 29.4) 1/4 inch thick which tapers to distally and it ends proximal to metatarsal head is fitted externally.

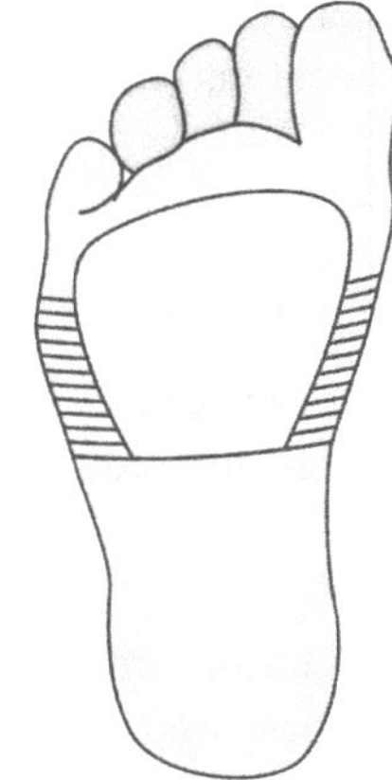

**Fig. 29.3:** Metatarsal pad : A detachable pad fixed inside the shoe to relieve pain on th metatarsals.

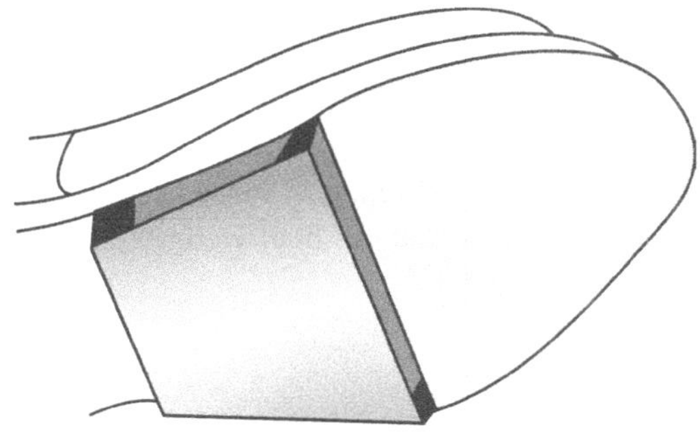


**Fig. 29.4:** Metatarsal bar : A rubber or wooden block placed outside the shoe to unweigh the metatarsals.

## • Heel Pain–Plantar Fasciitis

Plantar fasciitis is pain in heel due stretching of plantar fascia at anteromedial calcaneum.

a. Minor discomfort without hyperpronation of foot or high arch can be managed with
   i. Heel pad inside the sole of foot
   ii. Calcaneal bar placed distal to painful area
   iii. Scooped out cushion heel.
b. *Hyperpronated foot with decreased medial arch:* Custom made orthosis with subtalar joint in neutral position can be used.
c. *High arched foot:* An elevated arch support relieves heel pain.

## • Pain Behind Heel

Retrocalcaneal bursitis enthesopathy is the commonest cause of pain behind heel. It can be treated by raised heel thus reducing weight bearing and relieving pain.

## • Toe Pain

Pain in toe can be reduced by:

a. Extending the shark distally to reduce mobility of the joint
b. Metatarsal bar partly immobilize and reduce pain.

## • Limb Length Discrepancy

True length is measured from anterior superior iliac spine to tip of medial malleolus and apparent length is measured from umbilicus to tip of malleolus. True length may be normal but shortening may occur as a result of pelvic obliquity secondary to scoliosis or contractures. Limb length difference of ½ inch does not need correction. It is left for ground clearance. Up to 1 inch can be corrected by raising the insole. More than 1 inch can be raised with heel and sole.

## • Osteoarthitis of Knee

Foot orthosis can alter the ground reaction force thus useful in management for problems in proximal joints. Lateral heel wedge ¼ inch thick can reduce pain in OA with Genuvarum.

## Insensitive Foot

Loss of sensation can occur due to any lesion like:

a. Peripheral nerve lesion.
b. Spinal cord injuries.
c. Myelodysplasia

On weight bearing it may lead to:

1. Concentrated pressure over bony areas
2. Scarred plantar surface due to trauma
3. Bony deformity

For Concentrated Pressure

a. Microcellular insole to distribute weight over wide area.
b. Extra depth shoe.

For Scarred Plantar Surface

Any one combination of insole can be prescribed

a. Molded polyethylene foam backed by MCR
b. Molded poly ethylene foam with latex cork
c. Plastozole with or without added MCR.

For Bony Deformity

Deformity or ulceration over bony areas can be treated with soft molded insole of polymethane foam with areas of relief over bony areas.

- **Club Foot Boot**

Congenital talipes equino varus. Deformity has to be corrected by manipulation with strapping or by surgery. The corrected position can be maintained by club foot boot. The deformities in CTEV are corrected as follows:

*Equinus*

a. No heel in boot thus preventing equinus.
b. Front ankle straps that help to keep the heel down.

*Varus/Inversion*

Lateral border of foot is raised that keeps the foot in eversion.

*Fore Foot Adduction*

Medial border of the boot is made straight to prevent fore foot adduction.

- **Boots for Amputations**

a. Toe filler spacer in toe amputations.
b. Choparts boots in Chopart's amputation.

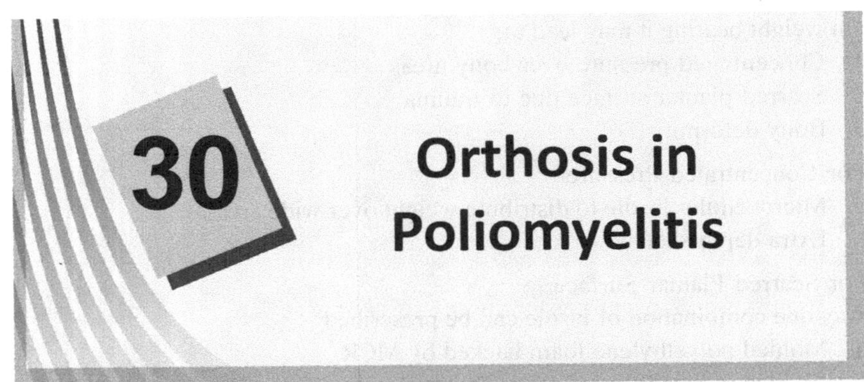

# 30 Orthosis in Poliomyelitis

Braces in polio were given in stage of recovery and in residual stage. All children with weakness in limbs should be advised to wear supportive orthoses until their growth is complete even if they are able to walk independently to prevent development of deformities. In adults decision on fitting of orthosis is based on a detailed clinical evaluation.

## CLINICAL EVALUATION

### Deformity

The common deformity in polio is:
Hip-flexion, knee-flexion, valgus and recurvatum, ankle and foot-Plantar flexion, calcaneal valgus and varus deformities.

Fixed deformities need to be corrected either surgically or conservatively by stretching, splinting, Wedge correction, etc. The corrected position is then maintained using orthosis. Mild degrees can be accommodated in orthosis.

### Shortening

Can be corrected by insole raise or by heel and sole raise.

### Muscle Power

Graded from 0 to 5.
Power of 3 or more in all group of muscles is considered adequate for independent Standing and walking.

## ORTHOTIC PRESCRIPTION

### AFO – Ankle Foot Orthosis

Prescribed for weakness in ankle and foot:

a. Free ankle is used when power is normal in ankle and foot
b. *Foot drop stop:* Weak dorsiflexors with equinus or foot drop
c. *Dorsiflexion stop:* Weak plantar flexion and calcaneal deformity.
d. *Limited ankle:* Ankle and foot flail. 10° dorsiflexion, 10° plantar flexion allowed.
e. *T strap:* Inside T strap for valgus deformity, outside or lateral T strap for varus deformity.

## KAFO – Knee Ankle Foot Orthosis

Used in weakness of quadriceps with or without weakness in ankle and foot. Isolated knee weakness can also be managed with knee cage. If the power of quadriceps is more than three KAFO is not necessary.

## HKAFO – Hip Knee Ankle Foot Orthosis

When hip abductors are weak and it can not stabilize hip, HKAFO with external hip joint and pelvic band is necessary.

## SPINAL SUPPORT

If spinal extensors are weak spinal support can be added.

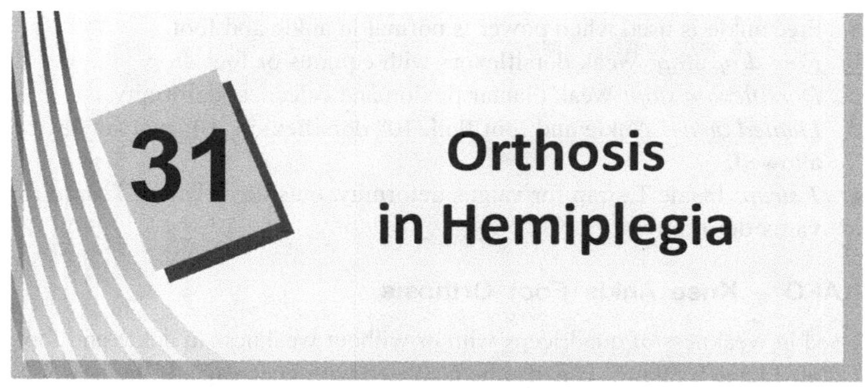

# 31 Orthosis in Hemiplegia

## LOWER LIMB ORTHOSES

The patient should possess the following before making him ambulant.

1. Ability to follow the instructions
2. Ability to maintain standing balance
3. Absence of contractures in hip, knee and ankle
4. Adequate return of voluntary power to stabilize hip at least in hip extensors as it stabilizes hip but also stabilizes knee.
5. Intact position sense in lower extremity (not an absolute requisite).

The problems in ambulation in hemiplegia is due to:

1. Motor weakness
2. Spasticity
3. Difficulty in ground clearance.

## KAFO

KAFO is given in hemiparesis patients with:

a. Knee instability with buckling or genu recurvatum
b. Ankle and foot instability with equino varus deformity. It consist of thigh band with metal bars with external knee joint with drop lock with anterior knee cap, calf band, ankle joint with 90° foot drop stop and outside T strap to control inversion with boot.

## AFO

Patients with spasticity in foot and ankle. It consist of calf band, metal upright, ankle joint with 90° foot drop strap with boot with outside 'T' strap.

## Cane

Lateral stabilization of hip is achieved by compensating the hip abductor by placing the cane on the opposite side.

## ORTHOSIS FOR UPPER LIMB

In common middle cerebral artery stroke, upper limb is more involved.

1. *Shoulder:* Shoulder slings are used to minimize shoulder subluxation. The different types of slings used are:
   a. Bobath sling
   b. Brewer kauper sling
   c. Common hemiplegic forearm sling
   d. Arm sling with humeral cuff and chest strap-does not restrict elbow movement (Fig. 31.1).

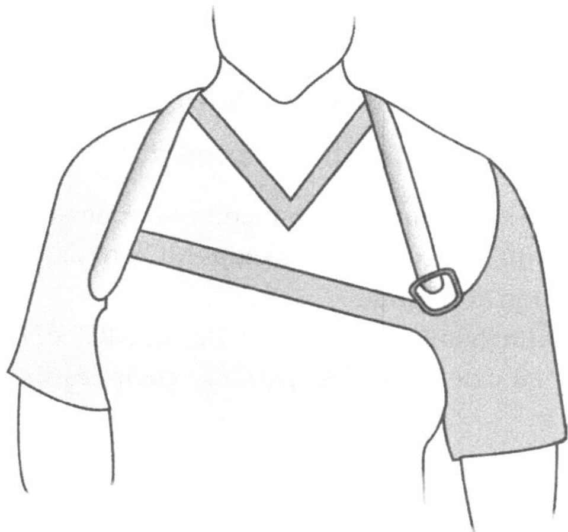

**Fig. 31.1:** Arm sling with humeral cuff and chest strap

2. *Wrist and hand:* Wrist and finger flexor contracture is the commonest deformity of upper links in hemiplegics. It not only increases the upper limb spasticity but also indirectly interferes walking by increasing lower limb spasticity. It is prevented by:
   a. *Pancake resting wrist hand orthosis:* It is a dorsal Wrist Hand Orthosis with wrist in dorsiflexion and extends up to interphalangeal joints to keep them in neural position, thumb in abduction and opposition.
   b. Dorsal cock-up splint.
   c. *Wrist hand cone:* Keeps metacarpophangeal joint in neutral position, thumb in abduction and fingers in minimal flexion.

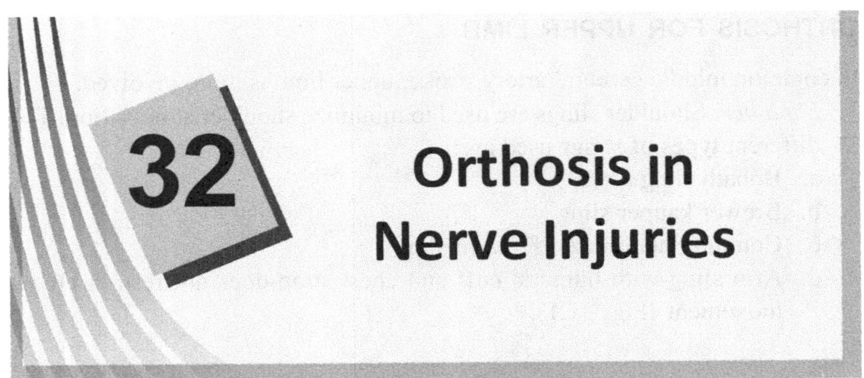

# 32 Orthosis in Nerve Injuries

## ORTHOSIS FOR MEDIAN NERVE INJURY

### Lesions at Wrist – 'Ape Tumb Deformity'

The orthosis aims to keep thumb in abduction or opposition position

1. Hand orthosis with "C" bar: "C" bar keeps MCP of thumb in abduction and allows free flexion at IP joint.
2. Hand orthosis with thumb post: It also holds the MCP of thumb in abduction but the distal end extends to and partially encircles the distal phalanx to stabilize it.

### Lesions Above Elbow

The deformity includes loss of wrist radial flexion, thumb flexion abduction and opposition and all finger flexion except ring and little finger.

1. The lesion is treated with wrist driven flexor hinge hand orthosis (vide dynamic upper limb orthosis).
2. Pointing index can be managed with strapping with middle finger (help flexion at DIP joint of index finger).

## ORTHOSIS FOR ULNAR NERVE INJURY

Ulnar nerve lesions leads to claw hand in little and ring finger with hyper-extension at MCP and flexion at PIP and DIP joints. It is due to weakness of lumbricals whose action is flexion of MCP and extension at PIP and DIP joints. But the long finger extensors which are supplied by radial nerve is intact. If the MP joints are kept in neutral or in 15° flexion, the long extensor can extend the IP joints.

1. Knuckle Bender Splint is a hand orthosis with lumbrical bar which keeps the MP joint in 15° flexion, thus allowing long extensors to act on IP joint.

2. Total Claw Hand is managed using a hand orthosis with MP block (lumbrical bar) over all digits is used (Fig. 32.1).

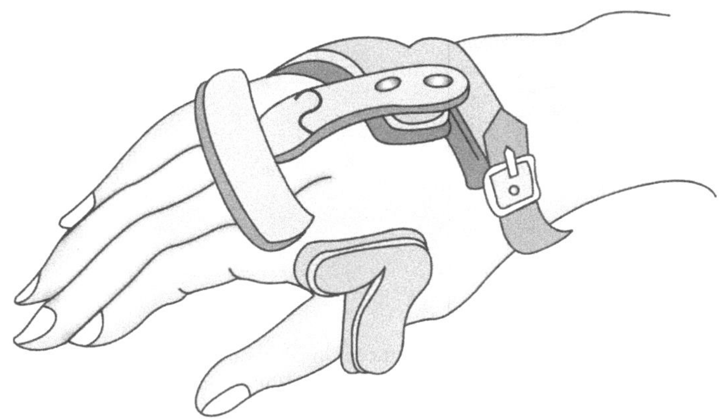

**Fig. 32.1:** Lumbrical bar

## ORTHOSIS FOR RADIAL NERVE INJURY

Injury to radial nerve results in wrist drop and finger drop. Posterior interosseous nerve injury leads to finger drop. The orthoses prescribed are:

1. *Static cock-up splint:* This keeps the wrist in dorsiflexion and it extends to keep the MCP joint in neutral position. Since it is only static splint, it prevents active movements.

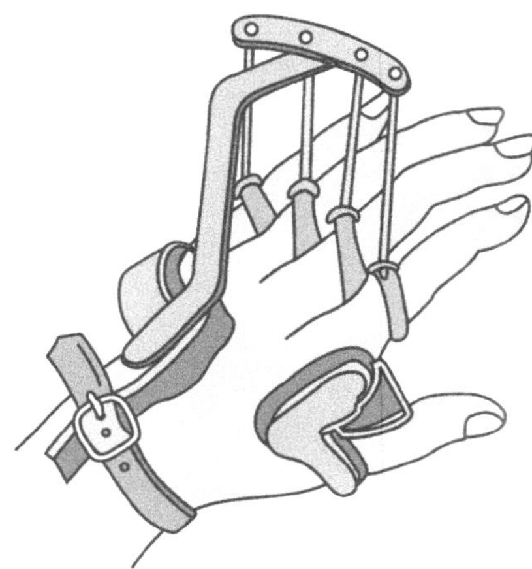

**Fig. 32.2:** MP extension assist

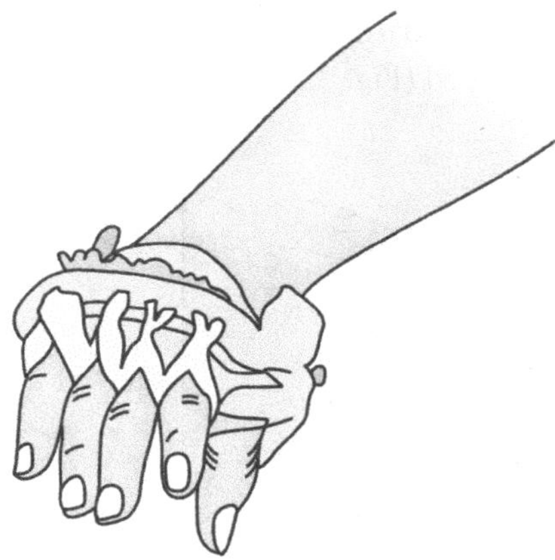

**Fig. 31.3:** Dorsal hand orthosis in posterior interosseous nerve injury (No wrist support)

2. Dorsal wrist hand orthosis with metacarpophalangeal extension assist: This keeps the wrist in neutral or dorsiflexed position with MP extension assist which is placed above proximal phalanx. The rubber bands are attached down to plastic finger piece to assist extension (Figs 32.2 and 33.3).

With good finger flexors, finger can be flexed. When released the rubber bands reposition the MCP in extension. PIP and DIP extension can be done by normal lumbricals. Instead of rubber bands springs can also be used for assisting extension.

With posterior interosseous nerve injury or recovering (wrist extensors power improving) radial nerve palsy, a dynamic MP extensor hand orthosis with MP extension assist without wrist support can be used.

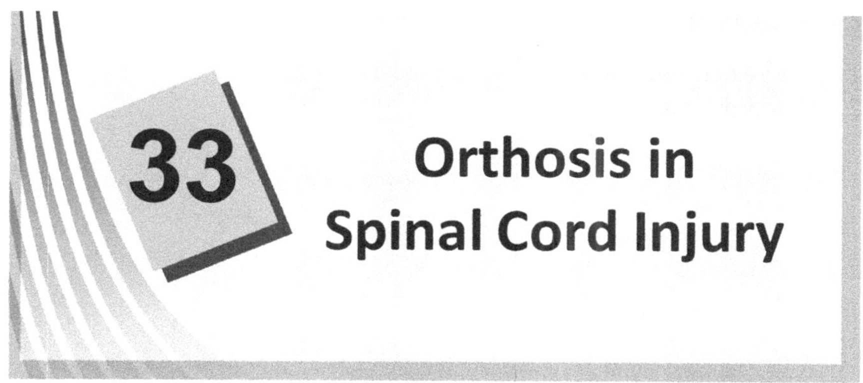

# 33 Orthosis in Spinal Cord Injury

Orthotic prescription in spinal cord injury patients depends mainly on the level of lesion.

## C4-5 INJURIES

1. Balanced forearm orthosis.

## C5 INJURIES (FIGS 33.1A AND B)

1. Over head slings
2. Long opponens orthosis
3. Electrically powered wrist extension flexor hinge reciprocal orthosis.

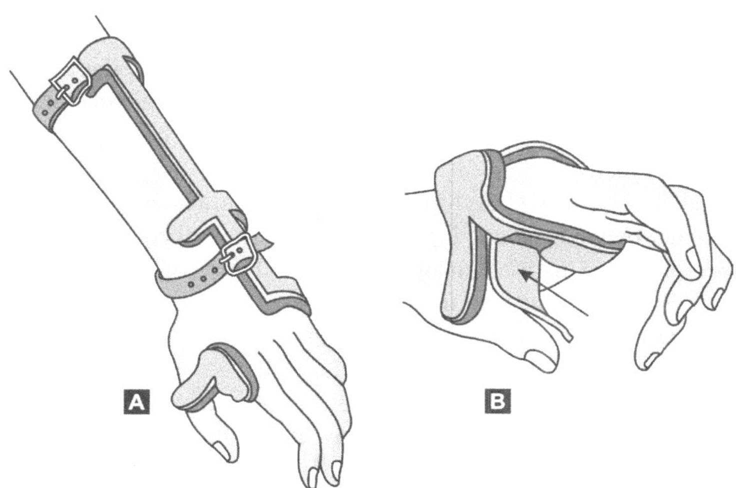


**Figs 33.1A and B:** A. Long Opponens Hand Splint: Maintains wrist in neutral position and fingers and thumb in functional position. B. 'C' Bar: An attachment that can be used in any hand orthosis to maintain thumb in opposition.

## C6 INJURIES

1. Wrist extension finger flexion reciprocal orthosis.
2. Short opponens orthosis.

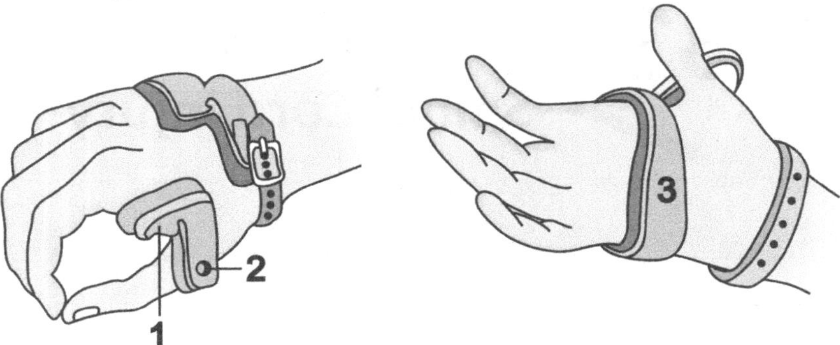


1. Radial extension 2. Thumb opposition 3. Palmar arch

**Fig. 33.2:** Short opponens splint maintains wrist in radical extension (corrects ulnar deviation), a opponens bar (thumb in abduction and internal rotation) and a palmar arch.

## C7-C8 INJURIES

1. Short opponens splint
2. Universal cuff

## LOWER LIMB ORTHOSIS

Number of orthoses are described in use for spinal cord injury patients.

1. *Bilateral KAFO:* It consists of medial and lateral uprights, upper and lower thigh bands, knee joint with drop lock, suprapatellar and patellar tendon straps, calf band, limited ankle and boot with microcellular insole
2. *Craigg scott orthosis:* It is a modified KAFO which is light weight and easy to wear.
3. *Conventional HKAFO:* Most paraplegics can achieve upright posture without pelvic band and hip joints. So it is prescribed only in high level paraplegics. The disadvantages of HKAFO are:
   a. Pressure ulcer over trochanter
   b. Difficulty in donning and doffing
   c. Ground clearance is difficult.
4. *Hip guidance orthosis/para walkers:* I is a modified HKAFO developed for paraplegics to lessen the energy expenditure. It consists of trunk band, pelvic band, hip joint, knee joint, and thigh and ankle cuffs. the patient stands with knee and ankle locked in neutral position. Ambulation is achieved by hiking the pelvis which allows the hiked leg to swing forward.

5. *Reciprocating gait orthosis:* It is also known as LSU brace. Developed in Louisiana state university. It is a modified HKAFO with a double Bowden's cable system that allows flexion in one limb and extension in the other limb.
6. *Advanced reciprocating gait orthosis:* It is a modified RGO where a single push pull cable is used instead of the double Bowden's cable.
7. *Isocentric reciprocating gait orthosis:* This is also a modified RGO where instead of Bowden's cable, a central pivoting bar and tie rod arrangement is given. This is more rigid and stable. It is beneficial for the patient as it causes less energy expenditure.
8. *Orthosis with functional electrical stimulation:* It is usually used with RGO.
9. *Floor reaction orthosis:* Vide foot orthosis.
10. *Ankle foot orthosis:* Vide foot orthosis.

Prescription of lower limb orthosis is usually as follows:

### Lesions at T1-T6

Not functional ambulators but can be tried with HKAFO with spinal support and a pair of axillary crutches. Patients normally do not use the orthoses.

### Lesions at T7 to T11

They become exercise ambulators in HKAFO with or without spinal support based on power of spinal extensors.

### Lesions at T12-L2

Have adequate spinal extensors and with KAFO with pair of axillary crutches, they may be able to walk for a short distance and can be domiciliary walkers.

### Lesions at L3-L5

AFO with or without elbow crutches. They have a good functional outcome and they become successful social walkers.

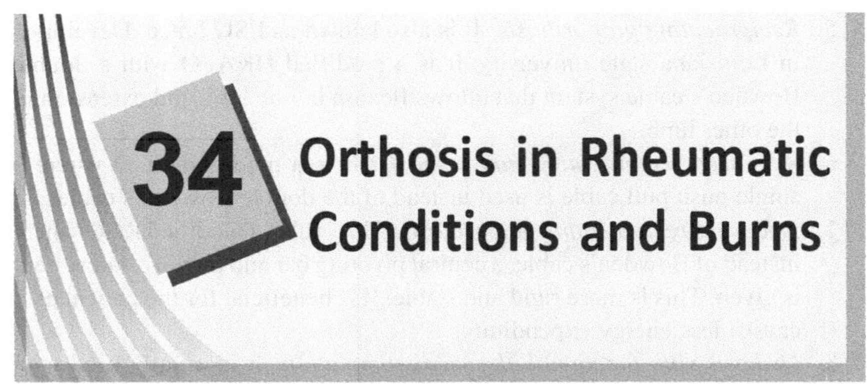

# 34 Orthosis in Rheumatic Conditions and Burns

## ORTHOSIS IN BURNS

1. *Early burns:* A static volar wrist hand orthosis with wrist in 15° dorsiflexion and MP flexion at 65° PIP and PIP in neutral position to prevent deformities.
2. *Axillary burns:* Air plane splints with shoulder in abduction and 20° forward flexion.
3. *Lower limb:* Resting splints in neutral position.

## ORTHOSIS IN ARTHRITIS AND SOFT TISSUE RHEUMATISM

Static splints helps to reduce acute inflammation.

1. Wrist hand orthosis in inflammation of hand.
2. Posterior static splints in lower limb arthritis.
3. *de Quervain's disease:* Thumb spica, wrist hand orthosis with wrist in neutral position and thumb radially abducted.
4. *Trigger finger:* Volar static hand orthosis to immobilize MCP joint in neutral position and allow full flexion in IP joint.
5. *Carpal tunnel syndrome:* Static wrist orthosis with wrist 0-15° extension.
6. *Swan neck orthosis:* Static dorsal PIP orthosis that prevents hyperextension at PIP joint
7. *Boutonniere orthosis:* Static volar PIP orthosis that prevents hyper flexion
8. *Ulnar deviation:* Dorsal hand orthosis with ulnar aspect MP block and individual finger stops.

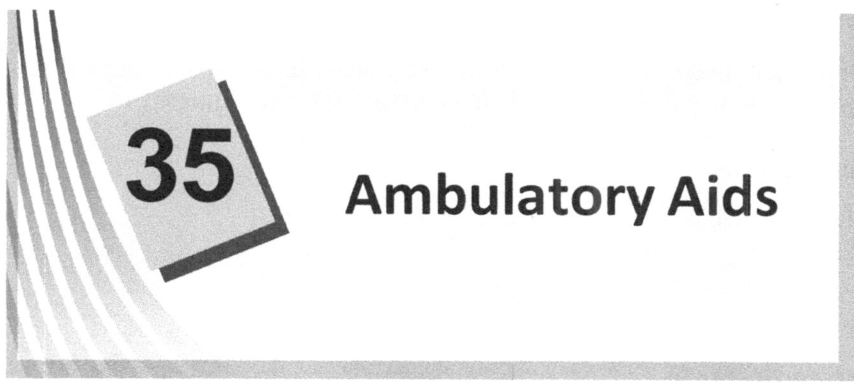

# 35 Ambulatory Aids

Ambulatory aids are devices which helps functional independence of patients by:

1. Increase the area of support thus maintaining the centre of gravity within support area.
2. Partially relieves weight.
3. Improve balance.
4. Reduce lower limb pain.
5. Provide propulsive force.
6. Provide sensory feedback.

The commonly used are (a) canes (b) walker (c) crutches.

## CANE

In unilateral cane weight transmission is around 20-25%.

### Indications

1. Painful conditions of knee, hip
2. Hemiparesis
3. Old age

### Measurement

Measured with patient in standing position from tip of cane to the level of greater trochanter.

### Types of Canes

1. "C" cane or J cane commonly used.
2. Functional grip cane provides more comfortable grip.
3. Quad cane or quadripod cane, provides increased area of support.

## WALKER

It provides maximum support for patient. It may be with wheels in front legs which help in patients with lack of coordination in upper limbs.

### Indications

1. Hemiplegia
2. Ataxia
3. Paraplegia
4. Cerebral palsy.

### Measurement

1. Place the front of walker 12 inches in front of patient.
2. Height is determined with shoulders relaxed and elbow flexed at 20° and measured from ground to wrist.

## CRUTCHES

### Types

1. Axillary crutches
2. Forearm crutches or orthoses
   a. Lofstrand crutches
   b. Evereh crutches
   c. Canadian crutches
   d. Platform forearm orthoses.

#### *Axillary Crutch*

Body weight transmission upto 80%.

*Measurement:*

1. *Crutch length:* Measured from anterior axillary fold to a point 6 inches lateral to fifth toe with patient standing and shoulder relaxed.
2. *Hand piece:* Measured with elbow flexed at 30° with wrist in maximal extension and finger forming a fist.

#### *Forearm Crutches*

Body weight transmission up to 40 to 50%.

*Lofstrand orthosis:*

- *Hand piece:* Patient standing shoulder relaxed with elbow 20° flexion with wrist in extension with fist.
- Proximal portion also angled at 20° for comfortable fit.

*Platform forearm orthosis:*
Indicated in:
1. Painful wrist and hand
2. Weak hand grips
3. Elbow contractures.

*Measurement:*
Standing with shoulder relaxed, elbow flexed at 90°. Distance from ground to forearm is measured.

*Evereh crutches and Canadian crutches:*
- Triceps weakness crutches
- Metal variety is known as evevh crutch and wooden is Canadian crutch
- These are like axillary crutches but it ends at mid arm level with a cuff. This prevents buckling (Flexion) of elbow during walking.

## Crutch Gaits

It depends on strength, balance, coordination, types of crutch and walking surface. The types of gaits are:
1. Two point gait
2. Three point gait
3. Four point gait
4. Swing to gait
5. Swing through gait
6. Drag to gait.

### *Two-point Gait*

*Sequence:*
1. Left crutch, right foot
2. Right crutch, left foot

It provides stability and is faster than four-point. It provides partial weight relief to both lower limbs.

*Indications:*
a. Ataxia
b. Decreased weight bearing in limbs.

### *Three-point Gait*

*Sequence:*
1. Both crutches
2. Weak lower limb
3. Normal lower limb

Also known as nonweight bearing gait.

*Indications:*
a. Lower limb fractures
b. Amputees

### Four-point Crutch Gait

*Sequence:*
1. Left crutch
2. Right foot
3. Right crutch
4. Left foot

Three points always in contact so good stability but slow in speed.

*Indications:*
a. Poliomyelitis
b. Ataxia
c. Paraparesis

### Swing to Gait

1. Both crutches
2. Advancement of limbs to the level of crutch.

### Swing through Gait

1. Both crutches
2. Advancement of both limbs past crutches.

### Drag to Gait

a. Alternate drag to gait:

*Sequence:*
- Left crutch
- Right crutch
- Drag limb to crutch level.

b. Simultaneous drag to gait

*Sequence:*
- Both crutches
- Drags limbs to crutch level.

# 36 Short Notes

## PROSTHESIS

1. Myoplasty
2. IPORD
3. 5 Day Hospital Rehabilitation Program
4. Childhood amputee
5. Neuroma
6. Phantom Pain
7. IPOP
8. Foot Amputations
9. Symes Amputation
10. PTB Prosthesis
11. Thigh Corset
12. Suction Suspension
13. Endoskeletal Prosthesis
14. Ischial Containment Socket
15. PTB SC SP or PTS Socket
16. Sach Foot
17. Energy Storing Foot
18. Quadrilateral Socket
19. Knee Disarticulation
20. Cat Cam Socket
21. NSNA
22. CAD/CAM
23. Gritti Stokes
24. Quadrilateral vs Ischial Containment Socket
25. Madras Foot
26. Indian Modifications in Prosthesis
27. Jaipur Foot

28. Vaulting
29. Drop Off
30. Abduction Gait
31. Medial or Lateral Whip
32. Harness
33. Elbow Hinges
34. Munster Socket
35. Slip Socket
36. Bowdens Cable
37. Hook
38. Voluntary Opening Hand
39. Voluntary Closing Hand
40. Figure of 8 Suspension
41. Extension Prosthesis

## ORTHOSIS

1. Dynamic Orthosis
2. Functions of Orthosis
3. Philadelphia orthosis
4. Thomas Collar
5. Peterson Orthosis
6. Somi Brace
7. Minerva Cervical Orthosis
8. Halo Cervical Orthosis
9. Lumbosacral Corset
10. Chair Back Lumbosacral Orthosis
11. Williams Brace
12. Taylors Brace
13. Jewett Orthosis
14. Boston brace
15. Milwaukee Brace
16. Air Plane Splint
17. Balanced Forearm Orthosis
18. Flexion Hinge Hand Orthosis
19. Wrist Extension Finger Flexion Reciprocal Orthosis
20. Long Opponens Splint
21. Short Opponens Splint
22. Cock Up Splint
23. Knuckle Bender Splint
24. "C" Bar
25. Ischial Weight Releiving Orthosis

26. Foot Drop Splint
27. Floor Reaction Orthosis
28. Functional Cast Bracing
29. Craig Scott Orthosis
30. Knee Cage
31. Reciprocating Gait Orthosis
32. Hip Guindance Orthosis
33. Arch Support
34. Thomas Heel
35. Metatarsal Pad
36. Metatarsal Bar
37. Insensitive Foot
38. CTEV Boot
39. Axillary Crutch
40. Forearm Crutch
41. Platform Crutches
42. Crutch Gaits

# Index

## D



## E



## F

## G

## L



## M



## N

## Q



## R



## S

## T



## U



## V



## W



## Y